About *The Fast Food Craze*

A childhood connection to animals led Tina Volpe to practice vegetarianism for more than three decades. Eventually she began to research the health consequences of eating on the run as well as the ramifications of fast-food advertising on our culture, home-life, and health, and on the present and future health of our children. Volpe's exploration of the fast-food industry also led to an examination of the treatment of animals within the U.S. agribusiness.

The Fast Food Craze contains the results of the author's research, as well as information for the reader on how to make conscious food choices that benefit one's health and support responsible farming practices. The dangers of a fast-food diet include risks posed by food-borne illnesses, along with increased risk of obesity, diabetes, cancer, and heart disease. Volpe explains current research in these areas and presents the reader with sensible alternatives—choices that bypass the skewed ad messages presented by profit-driven restaurants.

Vegetarianism is one option presented, but *The Fast Food Craze* is not primarily a call to abandon meat and poultry. It is a call to make conscious food choices for health and longevity. It is a call to hold corporations accountable for their impact on society. It is a call for the humane treatment of animals raised solely to satisfy our appetites.

Volpe presents evidence of the mistreatment of factory-farm animals; though raised to nourish us, in actual practice the reverse is true, as the very act of their exploitation harms our health and our spirits.

- Facts about Food-borne Illnesses
- Fat & Cholesterol Info
- Recommended Reading
- Related Web Sites
- Famous Vegetarians
- Health-conscious Grocers
- Related Not-for-profit Organizations

The Fast Food Craze

Wreaking Havoc on Our Bodies and Our Animals

Tina Volpe

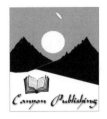

Canyon Publishing

Published by:
Canyon Publishing, LLC
12617 Trail Two
Kagel Canyon, CA 91342

www.fastfoodcraze.com

ISBN: 0-9761343-0-6
SAN: 256-2189
Library of Congress Control Number: 2005920341

Book Design: Janice M. Phelps

Cover photo by Derek Goodwin for Farm Sanctuary
Other photographs courtesy of :
FactoryFarming.org, Farm Sanctuary, and
United Poultry Concerns; used with permission.

Bulk purchases of this book are available to not-for-profit organizations. For information on such special orders, to order additional copies of this book, or for trade purchase order procedures, please visit www.fastfoodcraze.com or use the order form at the back of this book.

For Mom

To the animals I hear and see in my dreams,
I love each and every one of you,
and I am trying to get your voice heard!

Table of Contents

Introduction

Over the last nine to ten thousand years, or what has been documented anyway, most farm animals have been domesticated and dependent on human care . . . hence the term "Our Animals" in my subtitle. Animals have been mistreated and used for man's own selfish needs so obscenely over the years that it has become "our" responsibility to care for them and protect them. Factory-farmed animals are, at present, living the kind of life that mass murderers in prison couldn't even comprehend enduring. What have these precious animals done to deserve this? I know in my heart that this is wrong. My soul cries with them as they enter the slaughterhouses and listen to the screams of the others dying before them and the smell of the blood and the horrific machine sounds. Barbaric seems the only word that comes to mind, in a world where we can talk on telephone lines, use computers and travel to other countries in hours . . . Why can't we all realize how uncivil it is to treat other living creatures in this manner? If karma is truth, our world is going to have to pay its debt. I pray that *The Fast Food Craze* helps open your eyes and will reach down into your soul to actually find the compassion to see "our animals'" side.

Since I was a very small child, it has been my strong belief that we are not designed to eat the flesh or the many products derived from animals. Interestingly, most small children are naturally vegetarian. In my previous marriage, my ex-husband had three very small children at the time we were married, and in taking on the responsibility of raising them and feeding them, I recall each and every one of them disliked meat at an early age. Was this some sort of youthful intuition? Maybe because their minds and bodies had not yet succumbed to the major influence of society and the flood of advertising put out by the agribusiness? Perhaps because they are closer to the spirit of God, being so close to birth? Or is it just good old instinct? Whatever the reason, we can learn a thing or two from children.

The human body was not designed to eat animals. If we look back in history, many of the more highly intellectual and evolved humans who made a significant mark on this planet, suggest that living on a plant-based diet is the most healthy, humane and spiritually beneficial way to live your life. In the beginning, you will note in Genesis 1:29, "I have given you every herb bearing seeds which is upon the earth — and every tree in which is the fruit yielding seed; to you it shall be for meat."   This was the diet intended by God, in the perfection of the Garden of Eden.

Human beings do not have teeth capable of tearing flesh. We do not have the intestinal systems to warrant the process it takes to digest animals. If you look at at tiger, for instance, the teeth are meant to tear flesh. The intestinal tract is shorter and straighter than our human intestinal tract, therefore allowing elimination of the meat before fermentation, decay and rot takes place.

It is really very apparent, if you look at any of the diseases man has suffered over the years or the many health issues that are common today, they all relate to eating the flesh and/or products of another living, breathing, loving creature. What light has to come on for America to realize our world needs to awaken and see the truth?

My sister told me a story the other day about an acquaintance of hers who mentioned her husband was away on a hunting trip. The woman stated she would never eat the meat of the animal he shot and brought home . . . she couldn't endure eating a creature as cute as a deer . . . although, that very same day, she took her kids to McDonald's for hamburgers. Where did she think the meat came from that went into the meal her family consumed? It simply amazed me how little awareness was involved in this scenario. Do most people think that the burgers and nuggets that come from these fast food places, stores and restaurants actually just come from a scientists' lab or from the ground?

I wrote this book to help people like the McDonald's-diner woman realize that the deer that was shot in the forest (and I disagree with killing any animals) did suffer and die, however, there is no degree of suffering comparable to that of a factory-farmed animal — those same animals that get pushed into greasy burger patties, buffalo wings, chicken nuggets, eggs, milk, cheese, and every dairy product. These animals never knew what life was like in nature, never felt the dirt under their feet or felt the sunshine on their bodies, even just the simple, common everyday blessings that we take for granted, that God intended for them and gave them the right to enjoy . . . Bless their little hearts for what they went through to feed most of America and what they go through every second of every minute of every hour of every day.

I want to express to you the cries I hear in my dreams at night. The pigs that are begging to be saved and trying so hard to feel normal in such a wasteland of abnormality. The chickens trying to behave instinctively, but are screaming and going insane at the injustice of having their God-given rights taken away. The baby cows that cry out in the night, so lost, confused and lonely because they were ripped immediately from their mother's loving care, so that the human race can drink her milk, the milk that was intended for that baby cow. Are we insane? Or, is America just living in the darkest of ages?

I want to share with you that what I have learned writing this book I have found to be the most atrocious human unkindness ever bestowed upon another living creature. Sometimes I just want to cry of shame for what is being done to these beautiful, loving, kind and precious animals. What do you think they are thinking and feeling? These animals do have souls, so how can we possibly answer to them after they are gone or ever say we are sorry for putting them through such torture their entire life here on earth? How can we face our God when that time comes, knowing we are treating his creatures this way?

* * * * * *

When we think about fast food, what comes to my mind, is quick, easy and cheap. I realize this is very appealing to those who are financially challenged. The thought of our health sometimes doesn't come to mind . . . especially to the young. I know first-hand what it means to be in a hurry, and hungry and tired from working all day . . . however, is our health to be jeopardized so that we can have those few extra moments — moments that might be spent with the family finding and preparing meals that are actually nourishing and giving our bodies something with which to build and repair itself? When our bodies get fast food, it is getting nothing of the sort. No vitamins, no roughage, no live cells, nothing of value; what it is getting is a lot of things that are seriously doing damage . . . When, for the price of a couple of the child's meals at one of the large fast food chains, you can purchase a meal of fruit and veggies, whole grain breads, pastas and whole bean products that are actually going to do your body some good. Especially the fruit and veggies. There are a multitude of things you can do with just this food group, and quickly too! There are so many good cookbooks out there . . . and raw foods are the source of life to our bodies. The enzymes that are in raw vegetables and fruits are such a necessity to our cells and for our bodies to experience true health. My website (www.fast-foodcraze.com) gives many links to wonderfully healthy diets and plant-based cookbooks to get you started. Let's try, each and every one of us, to save some of these animals.

I hope that when you read this book, you find some helpful and enlightening information, and some compassion.

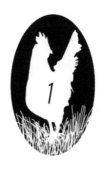

The fast food craze

"In 1970, Americans spent about $6 billion on fast food; in 2000, they spent more than $110 billion. Americans now spend more money on fast food than on higher education, personal computers, computer software, or new cars. They spend more on fast food than on movies, books, magazines, newspapers, videos, and recorded music—combined." -Eric Schlosser, *Fast Food Nation*

Total fast-food sales for 2003, $120.9 BILLION

In my youth, the fifties and sixties, I don't remember having many fast food restaurants available to me. McDonald's was around, but they were few and far between. For me, a peanut butter and jelly sandwich with an apple or a banana was a treat. (Which is probably why the cancer rates in those days were dramatically lower, and we didn't even know what obesity was.) What you are about to read may surprise, shock, and shake you to the core. It did me. I thought maybe, just maybe, I could help a little in this huge problem we have in America. Obesity, cancer, and last but certainly not least, animal cruelty.

The Fast Food Craze

What ARE we thinking?

Cancer rates have risen to the tune that one in four people are expected to contract some form of cancer in 2004. The statistics on nutrition-linked cancers is staggering. If Americans ate a healthy, balanced diet based mainly on vegetables, fruits, whole grains, and beans that help maintain a healthful weight, as many as one-third of all cancer deaths in the United States could be prevented. Numerous studies have demonstrated that dietary habits affect cancers at many sites. Strong scientific evidence has proven that diets high in fruits and vegetables have protective effects against cancers of the gastrointestinal tracts (e.g. colon, rectum) and respiratory tract (e.g. lung, larynx).

Diets low in fruits and vegetables have also been linked with increased risk of oral, ovarian, and cervical cancers. There is also evidence linking high-fat diets with increased risk of colon, prostate, and endometrial cancer. In 2003, about 556,500 Americans were expected to contract some type of cancer, that is a staggering 1,500 people per day. Cancer is the second leading cause of death in the U.S., exceeded only by heart disease. I truly believe both are attributed to America's obsession with fast food and its convenience. The poisons and chemicals in these products are all so nicely concealed. McDonald's and other fast food chains like Burger King have actually tried to add some healthier food options, like the veggie burgers, salads, and fruit. These efforts coincide with the ongoing threat of public and legal pressure. I believe this fast food craze is on its way out, if not by public awareness, by the lawsuits demanding that corporations label their "foods" for what they are . . . poison to our bodies!

The first McDonald's was built in 1940 by the McDonald brothers (Dick and Mac). McDonald's churns out an incredible volume and range of sophisticated propaganda. The company carefully targets sections of the population (parents, the media, health professionals, etc.).

Like many successful corporations, every marketing piece is very carefully written, to persuade, to motivate, to sell—not necessarily to clearly convey the facts. The success of McDonald's is dependent on its carefully manufactured image.

Of course it is *possible* to eat responsibly at McDonald's, as spokesmen for the chain never tire of reminding us. Fast food is simply one element of a balanced nutritional plan. Of course it's the *unbalanced* element, unless you order the fish filet sandwich with no mayonnaise, and one of those little salads with the lo-cal dressing; then you'll be fine, except for the filet being fried in beef tallow and full of saturated fat, the refined white flour in the bun and the high intake of sodium. Eating responsibly at McDonald's is a nearly impossible task.

In *Supersize Me*, a film by Morgan Spurlock, the producer decided to eat McDonald's food for thirty days, three times a day, and nothing else. This was brought on because of a television program Spurlock had watched about two teenagers from New York, who were suing McDonald's for making them obese. McDonald's responded by saying their food was nutritious and good for people. "Is that so?" Spurlock wondered . . . thus the McDonald's binge test was born. Taking a comic, yet serious look at America's addiction to fast food, Spurlock decided to make himself a guinea pig to find out the effects of fast food on the body. He ate McDonald's for one month, three times a day, and took a camera crew along to record it. When asked, he always "super sized."

Spurlock, thirty-three, was not prepared, nor were the three doctors who agreed to monitor him for this experiment, for the degree of ruin it would wreak on his body. Within days he was vomiting up his burgers and battling with headaches and depression. And, his sex drive vanished.

The doctors checked him regularly during the filming, as his weight ballooned thirty pounds, his blood pressure skyrocketed, his cholesterol went up sixty-five points, he endured symptoms of toxic shock to his liver, his skin began to look unhealthy, his energy dropped, he had chest pains, and his girlfriend complained about their sex life. At one point his doctors advise him to abandon McDonald's before he does permanent damage. They say they have seen similar side effects from binge drinkers, but never dreamed you could get that way just by eating fast food.

When the experiment ended, Spurlock's liver, from being overwhelmed by saturated fats, had virtually turned to pate'. "The liver test was the most shocking thing," said Dr. Daryl Isaacs, who joined the team to monitor Spurlock. "It became very, very abnormal."

Spurlock says, "I got desperately ill. My face was splotchy and I had this huge gut, which I've never had in my life . . . It was amazing and really frightening." In making this film, Spurlock traveled all over the country, and in all of his inter-views, McDonald's ignored his repeated requests for comments.

A recent lawsuit was filed against McDonald's, by a large vegetarian group, because they use beef tallow in their french fries, and yet told customers the fries were vegetarian. McDonald's apologized and agreed to settle the suit by paying $10 million, including $2.5–4 million to attorneys and $6 million to be allocated to various vegetarian groups (the "settlement allocation"). However, the fries continue to contain beef. McDonalds, after agreeing to pay these funds to "Vegetarian Groups," then misallocated the funds, some of which were directed toward anti-vegetarian groups and other groups that were set up to fight against vegetarian organizations.

In May, 2003 the final ruling was issued. McDonald's duped vegetarians twice, once when they lied about including animal products in their fries, and a second time when they promised to donate $6 million dollars to vegetarian groups, and then went on to convince the judge that black is white, and anti-vegetarian organizations are, in fact, vegetarian groups. "It's shameful," said one source close to the case. "It's as if they convinced the judge that you're kosher if you eat bacon." McDonalds would lose money if they didn't support the non-vegetarian groups and meat suppliers.

A friend of mine, who worked in the meat department of one of the major food store chains, told me a story of her experience with McDonald's. When McDonald's came to the store to purchase meat for their burgers, the store was turned down; their meat was not low quality/low priced enough. McDonald's went elsewhere.

Other fast food giants

Taco Bell was founded in 1962 and began franchising in 1964. The parent company, Yum! Brands, Inc. (previously known as Tricon Global Restaurants, Inc.), is the world's largest restaurant system with over 32,500 KFC, A&W All-American Food, Taco Bell, Long John Silver's and Pizza Hut restaurants in more than one hundred countries and territories.

Taco Bell has been under scrutiny due to its treatment of farm workers. Farm workers are among the lowest paid and most exploited laborers in the U.S. Average annual income for a farm worker is around $7,500.00, *per year.* Farm workers in the U.S. are boycotting Taco Bell, asserting that Taco Bell is huge in profits, at the injustice of the bent backs of farm workers.

As an example, Taco Bell is one of the largest buyers of Florida tomatoes. Since 1978, growers have paid the same piece rate, forty cents per bucket. That means that farm workers have to pick and haul *two tons* of tomatoes in a day to make $50.00. (Farm workers have demanded a one-penny increase on each bucket.) Workers are also denied the right to organize, to receive overtime pay, health insurance, sick leave, paid holidays, vacation or pension. In 2000, the Coalition of Immokalee Workers (CIW) made Taco Bell aware of these exploitive conditions, but they did not respond. A year later, the CIW launched a national boycott of Taco Bell, demanding that the multi-million dollar corporation recognize its role in exploiting farm workers and address the human rights violations in its supply chain. Since then, the Taco Bell Boycott has become one of the fastest growing movements for social justice in the country.

The CIW have received national recognition for their work drawing the links between corporate profits and farm worker poverty. In 2002, a caravan of workers crossed the country in the first Taco Bell Truth Tour, culminating in a massive march and rally at Taco Bell headquarters. Last year, seventy-five workers and allies held an unprecedented ten-day hunger strike outside Taco Bell's headquarters. This past year, November 2003, three CIW members received the 2003 Robert F. Kennedy Human Rights Award for their efforts.

As of July 2004, the workers and Taco Bell are still at an impasse. Taco Bell offered them a whopping $110,000, but the workers have not accepted it.

> Everyone knows this isn't the solution to the problem. The boycott continues. We will continue our campaign and it will keep growing. When they are really willing to solve the problem, we'll be willing to listen," coalition leader Rev. Noelle Damico of the Presbyterian Church (U.S.A.) said. "The consumer boycott is about the demands of Taco Bell and Yum!'s own customers who want the company to serve food that has been produced fairly, without the exploitation of human beings, beyond the moral imperative for the company to address known abuses in its supply chain. Yum! and Taco Bell should take this opportunity to gain a competitive edge on the market by being the first in the industry to serve fair food that respects human rights. *(For more information, visit www.pcusa.org/boycott)*

Taco Bell continues to spend upwards of 220 million on advertising, while lawsuits involving their own employees for wage violations exist. Taco Bell is also using genetically altered corn, not approved for human consumption by the FDA, in their taco shells. This corn was recalled by Kraft, Inc., however, Taco Bell chose to ignore the recall and continued using this corn in their shells.

Taco Bell continues to serve the lowest grade products obtainable — full of saturated fats and heaven only knows what else — which confirms my earlier statement . . . it's all about profits with these mega-companies, not serving us healthy meals.

In 1939, Colonel Harland Sanders first served the world, Kentucky Fried Chicken. Sanders invented what is now called "home meal replacement:" selling complete meals to busy, time-strapped families. He called it, "Sunday Dinner, Seven Days a Week." Today, Kentucky Fried Chicken, or as it is now known KFC, sells the equivalent of *736 million chickens annually.*

KFC Corporation, based in Louisville, Kentucky, is the world's most popular chicken restaurant chain. Every day, nearly eight million customers are served around the world. KFC has more than 11,000 restaurants in more than eighty countries and territories around the world. KFC is also a component of Yum! Brands, Inc.

On July 20, 2004, PETA (People for the Ethical Treatment of Animals) released the results of an undercover investigation into a KFC chicken slaughterhouse in Moorefield, West Virginia, where workers were caught on video stomping birds, kicking them, and slamming them against floors and walls. Workers ripped the animals' beaks off, twisted their heads off, spat tobacco into their eyes and mouths, spray-painted their faces, and squeezed their bodies so hard that the birds expelled feces.

The investigation was conducted at this location because it was the site of a KFC "Supplier of the Year" Award ceremony, and PETA wanted to see the "best" that a KFC supplier had to offer. This slaughterhouse is run by Pilgrim's Pride, the second-largest chicken company in the U.S., after Tyson Foods.

Animal-welfare experts are in agreement that the cruelty at this KFC supplier is reprehensible. Colorado State University professor of animal science, biomedical sciences, and philosophy, university distinguished professor, and university bioethicist Dr. Bernard Rollin writes, "I can unequivocally state that the behavior I saw exemplified in this videotape was totally unacceptable. ... The tape showed evidence of a work force that apparently failed to recognize that chickens are living sentient beings capable of feeling pain and distress." Dr. Temple Grandin, perhaps the industry's leading farmed-animal welfare expert, writes, "The behavior of the plant employees was atrocious," and asserts that even though she has toured poultry facilities in the U.S., Canada, Mexico, Australia, New Zealand, France, the Netherlands, and the U.K., the video showed "the WORST employee behavior I have ever seen in a poultry plant." University of Guelph professor of applied ethology and university chair in animal welfare Dr. Ian Duncan writes, "This tape depicts scenes of the worst cruelty I have ever witnessed against chickens. ... and it is extremely hard to accept that this is occurring in the United States of America." University of California at Davis School of Veterinary Medicine graduate and avian veterinarian Dr. Laurie Siperstein-Cook writes, "In NO case can the behavior of the workers be considered a necessary or acceptable way of killing or stunning chickens." (www.Peta.org)

PETA: Press Release

Hanover, Germany — Yum! Brands CEO David Novak, arriving in Hanover, Germany, to launch the first A&W Restaurant in that country, got a rude surprise when German animal rights activists, angered by the company's failure to reduce cruelty to chickens raised and killed for KFC, doused him in fake blood and stuck feathers on him, as others chanted, "Shame on you for cruelty to chickens." Mr. Novak was surrounded by bodyguards, but had separated from his entourage for a photo opportunity outside, which is when the activists made their move.

In the U.S., PETA has given up on negotiating with Novak and other Yum! Brands executives and has launched a vigorous campaign against the company's worst abuses of chickens. Among the improvements that PETA wants KFC to implement are the following: replacing crude and ineffective electric stunning and throat-slitting with contained-atmosphere stunning-to-kill; phasing out the forced rapid growth of chickens, which causes metabolic disorders and lameness; adding minimal enhancements, such as sheltered areas and perches; and implementing automated chicken-catching, a process that reduces the high incidence of bruising, broken bones, and stress associated with catching the birds by hand. PETA's recommended improvements are all approved by members of KFC's own animal-welfare advisory panel and are based on the latest available scientific research.

The campaign follows victories over McDonald's, Burger King, and Wendy's—all of which bowed to PETA pressure to reduce cruelty to animals raised and slaughtered for food.

"KFC stands for cruelty in our book," says PETA Director of Vegan Outreach, Bruce Friedrich. "There is so much blood on this chicken-killer's hands, a little more on his business suit won't hurt." Protests are planned in cities throughout the world and have already begun across North America, Europe, Asia, and Australia.

KFC recently ran an ad that seemed to suggest that fried chicken is the cornerstone of a healthy diet. Apparently, some people find this misleading.

The commercial begins with a "Lazy American Man" slumped in the living room in front of "The Game." In comes his slim and perky wife, who says, "Remember how we talked about eating better?" This causes Lazy Man to make a face. "Well," says the wife, "it starts today." Then she plops a twelve-piece bucket of chicken in front of him. An announcer quickly reels off various facts and figures suggesting that KFC's chicken is healthier than Burger King's Whoppers. Lazy Man, choking down another mouthful, removes any doubt among viewers that he's anything other than slow-witted by telling his wife that he's only doing this for her.

What is so amazing is that KFC has had to settle charges for this false advertising by the FTC (Federal Trade Commission), due to claiming that two chicken breasts have less fat than the Burger King Whopper. First of all, although it is true that two fried chicken breasts have slightly less total fat and saturated fat than a whopper, they have more than THREE times the trans fat and cholesterol, and more than twice the sodium, and more calories. The FTC will not tolerate any more of this false advertising. KFC Corporation also was charged for making claims that its fried chicken is compatible with certain popular weight-loss programs. UNTRUE. The settlement by the FTC and KFC will prohibit the company from making these or similar claims about the nutritional value, weight-loss benefits, or other health claims of its chicken products unless the company can substantiate the claims.

(For legal documents in this case, visit www.ftc.gov/os/ caselist/0423033/ 040603agree0423033.pdf)

Jack in the Box opened its first store in 1951, with a drive-through restaurant in San Diego, California. It started as San Diego Commissary, and later changed its corporate name to Food Maker.

Ralston Purina (yes, the dog food company) purchased a majority share in 1968 and started expanding, eventually buying the company outright in 1985. The name was changed to Jack in the Box, Inc. in 1999. Jack in the Box, Inc. also owns Qdoba Mexican Grill.

An article in the *Los Angeles Times* on January 24, 1993 reported the following: "A 2 year-old boy died Friday from a bacterial infection linked to tainted fast food restaurant hamburgers. The boy died of heart failure brought on by a kidney disease resulting from his infection with E. coli 0157:H7. At least 75 people, all in Western Washington, except for 2 in Spokane and 3 in Boise, Idaho have fallen ill from E. coli 0157:H7, this month. Most of those stricken were children who had eaten hamburgers at a Jack in the Box restaurant."

So began the ugliest, largest, and deadliest E. coli outbreak ever. Tragically, more than seven hundred people were made sick, dozens required dialysis, and four children died. The outbreak shattered the confidence Americans had in Jack in the Box. Jack in the Box was in crisis . . . It became synonymous with poisoned meat. Since the incident, to this day in fact, any article that discusses food-borne illnesses (E. coli, Mad Cow Disease, or salmonella) invariably mentions Jack in the Box. Jack in the Box is now a multi-million dollar company.

The fast food giants just keep getting richer, and they can afford to advertise. The natural food stores that many health-conscious customers frequent (Trader Joe's, Whole Foods, Full of Life, Follow Your Heart, and other such stores and restaurants) are never heard of in any real capacity. Although ABC recently ran a news report regarding the fact that the L.A. Unified School District now has a vegetarian menu added to their school's food choices. This was due to the efforts of animal rights advocates (PETA). It was a very short report; however, it was there.

Also, ABC ran another report about Chipotle's restaurant and healthy fast food using organic vegetables and animals that were not tortured in the factory-farm environment.

If animal rights groups and natural food stores were supported financially even at a small percentage of the amount of money available to the fast food giants, there would be much more awareness in commercials and other advertising. America is giving its hard-earned money to the fast food giants, and in return we are being unwittingly poisoned.

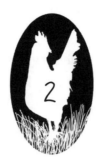

What are we thinking?

Let's face it . . . health is the single most important factor in our existence here on earth. If we don't have our health, we cannot enjoy life, period. So, let me just say that feeding the body correctly is essential to keep it working properly and to serve us on our journey in life with the least amount of failure. This can be done. But, it can only be done with the proper sustenance. Our bodies are fine-tuned machines and need to be treated as such. Giving it foods that do not nourish or detoxify our bodies is a waste and a detriment. It is frustrating to drive down the "main stretch" of many communities throughout the U.S. and witness the scores of fast food "restaurants," all brightly lit and beckoning. These food choices have no place in our communities, or our bodies, let alone our children's bodies. Can you imagine living on a diet of only fast food? Our bodies would be worthless after only a few months of this, yet we tend to lean toward these places because of convenience, and many families make these choices believing the "meals" to be a good value for their dollar. The following information may change your mind.

A pending lawsuit filed against fast food mega-corps McDonald's and Burger King may leave one of America's most beloved junk foods with a cigarette-like warning label: "May cause cancer."

Acrylamide, a chemical produced when carbohydrate-rich foods like french fries or potato chips are heated to very high temperatures, was discovered in 2002 by Swedish researchers to cause cancer and reproductive harm in high doses. Scientists in the UK, Switzerland, and Japan have all since reached the same conclusion. The FDA, along with the World Health Organization (WHO), considers acrylamide in food to be a "major concern."

Unsurprisingly, acrylamide is found in especially high levels in McDonald's' and Burger King's best-selling side order, french fries, which are cooked by both franchises at unusually high temperatures to achieve that admittedly yummy crisp. Problem is: the higher the temperature, the more acrylamide you ingest. According to an article in the *Guardian U.K.*, "Americans nowadays eat on average some 30 lbs of fries a year and . . . 35 micrograms of acrylamide a day—many hundreds of times what the WHO judges to be safe." These facts, and the lawsuit filed to publicize them, has the fast food giants concerned that sales of their high-profit products may plummet.

So how do all the new discoveries regarding fast food — the research into nutrition and health and the exposure of ingredients and nutritional benefits (or lack thereof) — affect the average consumer and their families? While no government or state agency seeks to pull the beloved french fry from the shelves, they all agree on one thing: Americans should be informed of the risks.

California's voter-approved Proposition 65 uses labels to "help consumers make informed choices about products," which let the buyer beware of chemicals in food and consumer products that are "known to the State of California to cause cancer, birth defects or other reproductive harm." Unfortunately for consumers, there is no practical enforcement of the rule.

Alan Hirsch, a spokesman for California's Office of Environmental Health Hazard Assessment (OEHHA), explains: "Acrylamide has actually been listed on Prop 65 since 1990, for the hazard associated with occupational uses of the chemical, but its presence in food has only been known for about two years. Labeling of chemicals on the list, although required, is not enforced."

That's precisely why McDonald's and Burger King are being sued. "Though it's the responsibility of individual businesses to have a warning for products on the list," Hirsch says, "Prop 65 allows any member of the public to enforce a warning if there isn't one in place." If the world's largest fry sellers lose, as many suspect they will, they'll be under court order to place acrylamide warnings in their California restaurants, if not directly on their packaging. Because fast food restaurants do about 60% of their business in the drive-through window, packaging labels may be preferred.

Enter Raphael Metzger of Long Beach, the tort lawyer representing the Council for Education and Research on Toxins (CERT) in the Prop 65 suit. "By targeting these two companies, the largest market share (of fry sellers) are represented. Addressing this issue with them means that the problem will be remedied in a large portion of the fast food supply, in foods that are highest in acrylamide." Currently, Metzger is waiting for the OEHHA to draft the language that will put people off their fries and chips.

From May 17 to 20, 2004, the National Institutes of Health convened a special panel to look specifically at the risks of acrylamide to reproductive health, ignoring its carcinogenic properties altogether. Though independent scientists found that there was a "minimal concern" that acrylamide levels could cause serious reproductive harm, chromosomal sperm damage was found in mice exposed to high doses of acrylamide (affecting the fertility of their offspring as well). The study concluded, however, that human reproductive health probably wouldn't suffer much damage.

"But," as the famous *Simpson*'s line goes, "what about the children?" In 1996, the Environmental Protection Agency recognized that children often metabolize chemicals and react to them differently than adults. According to Dr. Michael Shelby, Director of the National Toxicology Program at the Center for the Evaluation of Risks to Human Reproduction, "Kids get proportionately two to three times the level of exposure to acrylamide as an adult." Unfortunately, nobody has yet studied the effects of acrylamide on younger bodies, despite the fact that children are clearly targeted by the industry. Ronald McDonald anyone?

The Food and Drug Administration (FDA), whose aegis the issue falls under, has been studying acrylamide's affects on both cancer levels and reproductive health since the Swedish studies came out two years ago. Unsurprisingly, the embattled and increasingly pro-business agency has yet to release any data or warnings more specific than its ambiguous comment that acrylamide in food represents a "major concern." McDonald's, refusing to return phone calls, had no comment on the case or the studies.

SARS (Severe Acute Respiratory Syndrome): A deadly virus from the meat industry! For centuries, a province of China has had the world's largest concentration of humans, pigs and fowl living in close proximity. In this environment, pigs can become co-infected with both human and avian (bird) strains of influenza. When this happens, a deadly gene swapping can take place, in which the lethal viral strains can run rampant and the transmissibility of the human strains creates new mutated flu viruses capable of infecting and killing people on a global scale.

Other viral threats besides influenza have also escaped from Southeast Asian livestock operations. In 1999, a new virus, now known as the Nipah virus, jumped from pigs to humans in Malaysia, infecting pig breeders and killing about a hundred people before it was stamped out. In the Southern Chinese province of Guangdong, battery chickens are sometimes kept directly above pig pens, depositing their waste right into the pigs' food troughs. It may come as no surprise, then, that Guangdong is believed to be the beginning of the deadly SARS virus. The SARS virus is just the latest in a string of human tragedies traced back to our appetite for animal flesh.

According to the World Health Organization (WHO), SARS, which has already infected thousands worldwide, could become the "first severe new disease of the 21st century with global epidemic potential." And experts are again blaming intensive animal agriculture. According to China's equivalent of the Centers for Disease Control, the first people to succumb to the SARS virus were bird vendors and chefs, who had been in close and continued contact with chickens, ducks and other birds.

The concentration of animals with weakened immune systems in unsanitary conditions seems inherent to factory farming. As intensive livestock operations continue to spread worldwide, so will viral breeding grounds. Moving away from intensive animal agriculture and towards more sustainable plant-based methods of production may benefit the health of the planet and its inhabitants in more ways than we know. *(Source: World Health Organization)*

In June, 2003 the *CIDRAP News* reported: "Thousands of food handlers each year have hepatitis A and can potentially pass the disease to diners, a fact that poses tough problems for public health agencies, according to a report from the Centers for Disease Control and Prevention (CDC)."

About 230,000 cases of hepatitis A were reported in the United States from 1992 through 2001. Each year about 8% of adults who have hepatitis are identified as food handlers, indicating that thousands of food workers have the disease, the report says.

A food handler infected with hepatitis A virus (HAV) can potentially transmit HAV to many others and cause a substantial economic burden to public health.

There is also another health issue with regard to the fast food craze: Trans Fatty Acids (TFAs). TFAs are fatty acids that are formed when vegetable oils are hydrogenated, or partially hydrogenated, during the manufacture of fast foods, bakery goods, packaged snacks and margarine. TFA amounts are now required by the FDA to be listed on food labels, if applicable. The reason being that high TFA intake predicts an increased risk of coronary artery disease and diabetes.

Trans fats wreak havoc with the body's ability to regulate cholesterol. In the hierarchy of fats, the polyunsaturated fats that are found in vegetables are the good kind; they lower your cholesterol. Saturated fats, like those found in animal products, have been condemned as the "bad" kind. But trans fats are far worse. They drive up the LDL cholesterol, which markedly increases the risk of coronary artery heart disease and stroke. According to a recent study of some 80,000 women, for every 5% increase in the amount of saturated fat a woman consumes, her risk of heart disease increases by 17%. But only a 2% increase in trans fats will increase her risk of heart disease by 93%!

In 1999, the US FDA proposed that the Nutrition Facts labels on vegetable shortenings and some cookies, crackers, margarines, and other foods should carry information about trans fatty acids, or trans fats. In addition to requiring that some food labels list the amount of trans fats, the FDA rule would also define the term "trans fat free" and limit the use of certain nutrient or health claims related to fat content, such as "lean" and "low saturated fat."

In the realm of dietary dangers, trans fats rank very high. It has been estimated that trans fats are responsible for some 30,000 early deaths a year in the United States. Worldwide the toll of premature deaths is in the millions.

Texas Cattlemen vs. Howard Lyman & Oprah Winfrey

Source: International Vegetarian Union (www.ivu.org)

The verdict on the most recent appeal by "Cactus Feeders" against Oprah Winfrey and Howard Lyman, to a Federal Court has come in. The lawsuit against Oprah and Howard was "dismissed with prejudice." After almost six years and who knows how many millions of dollars in lawyer's fees, the case is over. Oprah and Howard won, and not only that, "Cactus Feeders," et al., are not permitted to appeal this verdict to a higher court (i.e., the Supreme Court) or pursue the matter anymore.

In April of 1996, Mr. Lyman (former cattle rancher) was invited to appear on Oprah to discuss Mad Cow Disease, food production, and the rendering process. He was part of a discussion of experts, including an expert from the beef industry, about food safety in the U.S. This included a discussion of potential health risks from E. coli and mad cow disease (which only weeks before was making headlines in Britain and throughout the world). When Mr. Lyman explained that cows are being fed to cows, Ms. Winfrey seemed to be repulsed by this thought, and exclaimed that it had just stopped her cold from eating another hamburger.

The show aired on a Monday, and beef futures—which had been in a steep decline due to drought, over-supply, and a number of complex factors—fell further on Tuesday. (Pundits referred to this as the "Oprah crash.") The cattle industry was apparently outraged, and pulled hundreds of thousands of dollars worth of TV advertising in retaliation. Pressured by television executives to mollify the cattle industry, Oprah offered to do an hour-long segment in which experts from the cattle business could debate

Mr. Lyman on her show. However, the cattlemen refused to appear on the show if Lyman were going to be present. They did not desire such a debate.

So, Oprah subsequently permitted a cattle business "expert" to appear and speak for ten minutes on her show, presenting the meat industry "side" in which the meat industry could say whatever they wished, secure in the knowledge that no opposing or questioning viewpoint would be heard.

A short time later, some Texas cattlemen, led by billionaire Paul Engler, owner of Cactus Feeders, Inc., filed suit against Lyman, Oprah, Harpo Productions (which produces Oprah) and King World Syndicator (King World was released from the suit by summary judgment). The lawsuit alleged Lyman and Oprah had violated a Texas law, which forbids someone from "knowingly making false statements" about agricultural business. The cattlemen have alleged that Oprah is responsible for the decline in beef futures.

The unprecedented trial took place in Amarillo, Texas—right in the middle of cattle ranching country, from where the jury has been selected—despite numerous requests from the defendants to move the trial to another part of Texas.

On February 29, 1998, the Texas jury found then Humane Society of the U.S. Program Director Howard Lyman and Oprah Winfrey not liable for comments made on the national show about eating beef.

Mr. Lyman, now the President of Voice for a Viable Future, spent six weeks in Amarillo fighting "food disparagement" and libel charges against him. Until the jury rendered its judgment, Lyman and associates were barred from speaking about the lawsuit as a result of a court-imposed gag order.

Lyman, who spent much of his professional life raising cattle, has been traveling the globe year-round since 1991, speaking on health, environment, and animal issues, stated:

> Today . . . I breathe more easily, knowing that a vigorous debate about potential dangers to our food supply—ranging from E. coli to pfiesteria to salmonella to mad cow disease—is permissible. Lawsuits like this stifle speech about matters that have implications for the health and welfare of every American consumer. At a time when threats to food safety are arguably greater than ever—threats exacerbated by intense confinement conditions that abet the spread of disease, and by controversial feeding practices—we need a free and open discussion about these matters.

The battle isn't over. Thirteen states, including Texas, have passed laws designed to silence and intimidate those who expose unsafe and unhealthy factory farm and slaughterhouse practices. These so-called "food disparagement" laws make it a crime to criticize food and how it is produced.

In Britain, twenty-two people died from Mad Cow disease. In the U.S., over 9,000 deaths occur yearly due to food-borne illnesses such as E. coli. Unsafe food is deadly. It is time to challenge these laws. It is time to stand up to those who put their own economic interests above the public's safety.

Within a few months after the Oprah show aired and caused a firestorm of controversy, the Food and Drug Administration announced pending regulations to eliminate the feeding of ruminants to ruminants. The specific content of the regulations were delayed until after the presidential elections of 1996, most likely to avoid offending the live-stock industry. Finally, the August 1997 ban on feeding ruminants to ruminants, a necessary but insufficient measure to stave off the spread of mad cow disease to America, went into effect.

U.S. Continues to Violate World Health Organization Guidelines for BSE (Mad Cow Disease)

(World Health Organization website: www.who.int/en/)

January 23, 2004 Michael Greger, M.D. for the Organic Consumers Association: The United States is violating all four concrete recommendations laid down by the World Health Organization to prevent the spread of BSE (Bovine Spongiform Encephalopathy), or mad cow disease, into the human population. Inadequate testing of the brains of U.S. cattle is likely missing hundreds of cases of BSE and inade-quate testing of the brains of human dementia victims is likely missing hundreds of cases of the human spongiform encephalopathy, sporadic Creutzfeldt Jakob disease. New research suggests that some of these cases of the sporadic form of CJD may be caused by eating BSE-infected meat. Until we follow the guidelines set forth by the World Health Organization and the Food and Agriculture Organization of the United Nations and enact science-based safeguards proven to work in Europe—such as a total ban on the feeding of slaughterhouse waste, blood and excrement to farmed animals, and dramatically increased surveillance for both these diseases-the safety of the American food supply will remain in question.

WHO Recommendation #1:
Stop Feeding Infected Animals to Other Animals

The number one recommendation of the World Health Organization was that no "part or product" of any animal showing signs of a transmissible spongiform encephalopathy (TSE), or mad cow-like disease, should be fed to any animal. "All countries," the guideline reads, "must ensure the slaughter and safe disposal of TSE-affected animals so that TSE infectivity cannot enter any food chain." Yet, in the U.S., it remains legal to feed deer and elk known to be infected with a transmissible spongiform encephalopathy called chronic wasting disease (CWD)—and to feed downer cows untested for Mad Cow disease—to livestock such as pigs and chickens.

Although science has yet to investigate whether pigs and chickens are susceptible to "mad deer" prions, there is a concern that even if these animals don't develop clinical symptoms of the disease, they could become so-called "silent carriers." Dr. Richard Race is a Senior Investigator with the National Institutes of Health. In 2001, he published a landmark paper showing that even species thought to be resistant to particular strains of prions could invisibly harbor the disease and pass it on to other animals. He also found that these deadly prions were somehow able to adapt to the new species, becoming even more lethal and replicating faster and faster.

Dateline NBC quoted D. Carleton Gajdusek, the first to be awarded a Nobel Prize in Medicine for his work on prion diseases as saying, "It's got to be in the pigs as well as the cattle. It's got to be passing through the chickens." Dr. Paul Brown, medical director for the U.S. Public Health Service, believes that pigs and poultry could indeed be harboring mad cow disease and passing it on to humans, adding that pigs are especially sensitive to the disease. "It's specula-tion," he says, "but I am perfectly serious."

At a 2002 symposium on chronic wasting disease, Dr. Race expressed concern that U.S. cattle could be invisibly harboring the chronic wasting disease seen in wildlife and passing it on to humans. The reason Dr. Race is so concerned is because chronic wasting disease seems unique in that it's the only prion disease thought to be spread by casual contact through exposure to, or exchange of, bodily fluids such as saliva. And the best available research suggests that CWD prions can infect humans as well, perhaps even as readily as Mad Cow prions. Dr. Race wonders if people could also become silent carriers. And, "If these people are subclinical carriers," Race asked, "do they represent a threat to other people?" All transmissible spongiform encephalopathies are invariably fatal. Consumer advocates argue that these prions should not be allowed to enter the food chain.

In May 2003, the Food and Drug Administration finally drafted proposed voluntary "suggestions" for the rendering industry, recommending that deer and elk infected with chronic wasting disease, or at high risk for the disease, be excluded from animal feed. However, even if this proposal were enacted, it would represent only non-binding, non-enforceable "guidance" recommendations for the industry. The FDA made these same kinds of "guidance" recommen-dations to pharmaceutical companies over a decade ago, discouraging the use of bovine-derived materials from coun-tries with mad cow disease in manufacturing their vaccines, only to learn seven years later that major pharmaceutical manufacturers simply ignored the recommendations.

Europe's Scientific Steering Committee met in 2003 and agreed that the U.S. should comply with the World Health

Organization guidelines and ban the feeding of animals infected with chronic wasting disease to other animals. The United States seems to be the only country that still legally allows prion-infected animals to be fed to other animals, including to those animals destined for the dinner plate.

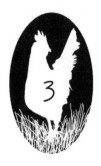

The animals on our plates

"All beings tremble before violence. All fear death. All love life."
-Buddha

"The greatness of a nation and its moral progress can be judged by
the way its animals are treated."
-M. Gandhi

"The more I have learned, the more I have felt that if people knew
what really goes on they would make major changes in their food
choices. Major changes that would go a very long way, not only
towards improving their own health, but towards reducing the
suffering in the world as well."
-John Robbins, *Diet for a New America*

The Fast Food Craze

"Although other animals cannot reason or speak the way humans do, this does not give us the right to do with them as we like. Even though our supposed possession of a soul and superior intelligence are used to create an arbitrary dividing line over rights, the fact remains that all animals have the capacity to experience pain and suffering, and in suffering they are our equals.
— Nathaniel Altman (1948-)

"The earth is the Lord's and the fullness Thereof, Oh, God, enlarge within us the Sense of fellowship with all living Things, our brothers the animals to Whom Thou gavest the earth as Their home in common with us ... May we realize that they live not For us alone but for themselves and For Thee and that they love the sweetness Of life."
— St. Basil, Bishop of Caesarea (330-379)

"The old assumption that animals acted exclusively by instinct, while man had a monopoly of reason, is, we think, maintained by few people nowadays who have any knowledge at all about animals. We can only wonder that so absurd a theory could have been held for so long a time as it was, when on all sides the evidence of animals' power of reasoning is crushing."
— Ernest Bell (1851-1933)

The animals on our plates

"The day may come when the rest of the animal creation may acquire those rights which never could have been withheld from them but by the hand of tyranny . . . a full-grown horse or dog is beyond comparison a more rational, as well as a more conversable animal, than an infant of a day, or a week or even a month old. But suppose the case were otherwise, what would it avail? The question is not, can they reason? Nor, can they talk? But, can they suffer? Why should the law refuse its protection to any sensitive being? The time will come when humanity will extend its mantle over everything which breathes. . . ."
– Jeremy Bentham (1748-1832)

"We find amongst animals, as amongst men, power of feeling pleasure, power of feeling pain; we see them moved by love and by hate; we see them feeling terror and attraction; we recognize in them powers of sensation closely akin to our own, and while we transcend them immensely in intellect, yet in mere passional characteristics our natures and the animals' are closely allied. We know that when they feel terror, that terror means suffering. We know that when a wound is inflicted, that wound means pain to them. We know that threats bring to them suffering; they have a feeling of shrinking, of fear, of absence of friendly relations, and at once we begin to see that in our relations to the animal kingdom a duty arises which all thoughtful and compassionate minds should recognize—the duty that because we are stronger in mind than the animals, we are or ought to be their guardians and helpers, not their tyrants and oppressors, and we have no right to cause them suffering and terror merely for the gratification of the palate, merely for an added luxury to our own lives."
– Annie Besant (1847-1933)

The Fast Food Craze

"What the factory farmers emphasize is that animals are different
from humans: we can't, we are told, judge their reactions by our
own, because they don't have human feelings. But no one in his
senses ever supposed they did. Anyone acquainted with animals can
guess pretty well that they have less intellect and memory than
humans, and live closer to their instincts. But the reasonable conclusion to draw from this is the very opposite of the one the factory
farmers try to force upon us. In all probability, animals feel more
sharply than we do any restrictions on such instinctual promptings
as the need, which we share with them, to wander around and
stretch one's legs every now and then; and terror or distress
suffered by an animal is never, as sometimes in us, softened by
intellectual comprehension of the circumstances."
– Brigid Brophy (1929-)

"On profit-driven factory farms, veal calves are confined to dark
wooden crates so small that they are prevented from lying down
or scratching themselves. These creatures feel; they know pain.
They suffer pain just as we humans suffer pain. Egg-laying hens are
confined to battery cages. Unable to spread their wings, they are
reduced to nothing more than an egg-laying machine. . . . The law
clearly requires that these poor creatures be stunned and rendered
insensitive to pain before [the slaughtering] process begins. Federal
law is being ignored. Animal cruelty abounds. It is sickening. It is
infuriating. Barbaric treatment of helpless, defenseless creatures
must not be tolerated even if these animals are being raised for
food—and even more so, more so. Such insensitivity is insidious and
can spread and is dangerous. Life must be respected and dealt with
humanely in a civilized society."
– Senator Robert Byrd (on the floor of the U.S. Senate,
July 9, 2001)

The animals on our plates

"Never believe that animals suffer less than humans. Pain is the same for them that it is for us. Even worse, because they cannot help themselves."
— Dr. Louis J. Camuti (1893-1981)

"The saints are exceedingly loving and gentle to mankind, and even to brute beasts . . . . Surely we ought to show [animals] great kindness and gentleness for many reasons, but, above all, because they are of the same origin as ourselves."
— St. John Chrysostom (347-407)

"There is no fundamental difference between man and the higher mammals in their mental faculties. . . . The difference in mind between man and the higher animals, great as it is, certainly is one of degree and not of kind. The love for all living creatures is the most noble attribute of man. We have seen that the senses and intuitions, the various emotions and faculties, such as love, memory, attention and curiosity, imitation, reason, etc., of which man boasts, may be found in an incipient, or even sometimes a well-developed condition, in the lower animals."
— Charles Darwin (1809-1882)

The Fast Food Craze

"To my mind, the life of a lamb is no less precious than that of a
human being. I should be unwilling to take the life of a lamb for the
sake of the human body. I hold that, the more helpless a creature,
the more entitled it is to protection by man from the cruelty of
man. . . . I want to realize brotherhood or identity not merely with
the beings called human, but I want to realize identity with all life,
even with such things as crawl upon earth."
– Mahatma Gandhi (1869-1948)

"This [eating animals] appears from the frequent hardheartedness
and cruelty found among those persons whose occupations engage
them in destroying animal life, as well as from the uneasiness
which others feel in beholding the butchery of animals. It is most
evident in respect to the larger animals and those with whom we
have a familiar intercourse—such as oxen, sheep, and domestic fowls,
etc. They resemble us greatly in the make of the body, in general,
and in that of the particular organs of circulation, respiration, diges-
tion, etc.; also in the formation of their intellects, memories and
passions, and in the signs of distress, fear, pain, and death. They
often, likewise, win our affections by the marks of peculiar sagacity,
by their instincts, helplessness, innocence, nascent benevolence, etc.,
and if there be any glimmering hope of an 'hereafter' for them—if
they should prove to be our brethren and sisters in this higher
sense—in immortality as well as mortality, in the permanent prin-
ciple of our minds as well as in the frail dust of our bodies—this
ought to be still further reason for tenderness for them."
– David Hartley (1705-1757)

The animals on our plates

"The soul is the same in all living creatures, although the body of
each is different."
– Hippocrates (460--370 BC)

"I have from an early age abjured the use of meat, and the time will
come when men such as I will look upon the murder of animals as
they now look upon the murder of men."
– Leonardo da Vinci (1452-1519)

"It should not be believed that all beings exist for the sake of the
existence of man. On the contrary, all the other beings too have
been intended for their own sakes and not for the sake of anything
else ... there is no difference between the pain of humans and the
pain of other living beings, since the love and tenderness of the
mother for the young are not produced by reasoning, but by feeling,
and this faculty exists not only in humans but in most living beings."
– Rabbi Moses ben Maimon (1135-1204)

"Since factory farming exerts a violent and unnatural force upon the
living organisms of animals and birds in order to increase production and profits; since it involves callous and cruel exploitation of
life, with implicit contempt for nature, I must join in the protest
being uttered against it. It does not seem that these methods have
any really justifiable purpose, except to increase the quantity of
production at the expense of quality—if that can be called a
justifiable purpose."
– Thomas Merton (1915-1968)

The Fast Food Craze

"But for the sake of some little mouthful of flesh we deprive a soul
of the sun and light, and of that proportion of life and time it had
been born into the world to enjoy."
– Plutarch (in Moralia) (46-120)

"The welfare of animal citizens is as much our concern as is that of
other humans. Surely if we are all God's creatures, if all animal
species are capable of feeling, if we are all evolutionary relatives, if
all animals are on the same biological continuum, then also we
should all be on the same moral continuum—and if it is wrong to
inflict suffering upon an innocent and unwilling human, then it is
wrong to so treat another species."
– Richard D. Ryder (1940-)

"The emancipation of men from cruelty and injustice will bring with
it in due course the emancipation of animals also. The two reforms
are inseparably connected, and neither can be fully realized alone."
– Henry Salt (1851-1939)

"If the use of animal food be, in consequence, subversive to the
peace of human society, how unwarrantable is the injustice and the
barbarity which is exercised toward these miserable victims. They
are called into existence by human artifice that they may drag out
a short and miserable existence of slavery and disease, that their
bodies may be mutilated, their social feelings outraged. It were
much better that a sentient being should never have existed, than
that it should have existed only to endure unmitigated misery."
– Percy Bysshe Shelley (1792-1822)

The animals on our plates

"The same questions are bothering me today as they did fifty years ago. Why is one born? Why does one suffer? In my case, the suffering of animals also makes me very sad. I'm a vegetarian, you know. When I see how little attention people pay to animals, and how easily they make peace with man being allowed to do with animals whatever he wants because he keeps a knife or a gun, it gives me a feeling of misery and sometimes anger with the Almighty. I say 'Do you need your glory to be connected with so much suffering of creatures without glory, just innocent creatures who would like to pass a few years in peace?' I feel that animals are as bewildered as we are except that they have no words for it. I would say that all life is asking: 'What am I doing here?'"
– Isaac Bashevis Singer, Newsweek interview (October 16, 1978) after winning the Nobel Prize in literature.

"How pitiful, and what poverty of mind, to have said that the animals are machines deprived of understanding and feeling ... has Nature arranged all the springs of feeling in this animal to the end that he might not feel? Has he nerves that he may he incapable of suffering? People must have renounced, it seems to me, all natural intelligence to dare to advance that animals are but animated machines ... It appears to me, besides, that [such people] can never have observed with attention the character of animals, not to have distinguished among them the different Voices of need, of suffering, of joy, of pain, of love, of anger, and of all their affections. It would be very strange that they should express so well what they could not feel. ... They are endowed with life as we are, because they have the same principles of life, the same feelings, the same ideas, memory, industry—as we."
– Voltaire (1694-1778)

Excerpts from an Interview
with Cardinal Ratzinger

by German journalist Peter Seewald

Cardinal Ratzinger is the Prefect for the Congregation for the Doctrine of the Faith, the Vatican's foremost advisor on matters of doctrine.

Seewald: Are we allowed to make use of animals, and even to eat them?

Ratzinger: That is a very serious question. At any rate, we can see that they are given into our care, that we cannot just do whatever we want with them. Animals, too, are God's creatures, and even if they do not have the same direct relation to God that man has, they are creatures of his will, creatures we must respect as companions in creation and as important elements in the creation.

As far as whether we are allowed to kill and to eat animals, there is a remarkable ordering of matters in Holy Scripture. We can read how, at first, only plants are mentioned as providing food for man. Only after the flood, that is to say, after a new breach has been opened between God and man, are we told that man eats flesh . . . Nonetheless . . . we should not proceed from this to a kind of sectarian cult of animals. For this, too, is permitted to man. He should always maintain his respect for these creatures, but he knows at the same time that he is not forbidden to take food from them. Certainly, a sort of industrial use of creatures, so that geese are fed in such a way as to produce as large a liver as possible, or hens live so packed together that they become just caricatures of birds, this degrading of living creatures to a commodity seems to me in fact to contradict the relationship of mutuality that comes across in the Bible.

Celebrity Quotes
Famous Friends of Farm Sanctuary Quotes:

"I think people will be shocked to find that most of the meat they eat as consumers, whether it be in fast food or even at your supermarket, is coming from animals that live most of their lives in stress and fear."
— Noah Wyle, Actor

"We can no longer deny that farm animals are living, breathing, sentient creatures who deserve to be treated humanely and need protection under the law."
— Mary Tyler Moore, Actress

"If anyone wants to save the planet, all they have to do is just stop eating meat. That's the single most important thing you could do. It's staggering when you think about it. Vegetarianism takes care of so many things in one shot: Ecology, famine, cruelty"
— Sir Paul McCartney

"If any kid ever realized what was involved in factory farming they would never touch meat again. I was so moved by the intelligence, sense of fun and personalities of the animals I worked with on Babe that by the end of the film I was a vegetarian."
— James Cromwell, Actor

"The question, as my friend Debby Tanzer says, is not whether animals should have rights, but what gives us the right to slaughter, what gives us the right?"
— Sue Coe, Artist

"It's really important to counteract the corporate propaganda that kids get about meat, dairy, eggs and how animals are treated generally. It's important to expose kids to another kind of message."
— Casey Affleck.

The Fast Food Craze

"If we were to be eating chicken this evening — my little crib sheet says to remind everybody — that by serving 360 people this evening we would be killing 120 chickens at this meal alone. And if they were factory farmed, they are animals who would have lived in a stressful condition for their entire existence. And if we are what we eat, we should be careful."
— Stefanie Powers, Actress

"We have a lot of work ahead of us. We consider ourselves a compassionate society and yet we don't show compassion to the very beings that we share the planet with. That has to change."
— Gary Ackerman, U.S. Representative

"Farm animal cruelties are often ignored, even gross neglect such as starvation and abandonment. Severe cruelty cases involving cattle, pigs, chickens and other farm animals are seldom prosecuted and the animals are generally left to suffer and die or sent to auctions or slaughterhouses."
— Linda Blair, Actress

"There are viable (and usually better) alternatives to the use of animals for food, sport, clothing, and experimentation. I beg you to discontinue any actions that might cause or condone animal torture, abuse, or destruction."
— Moby, Musician

"I am against killing and cruelty. That's why I'll always be a tofu and potatoes man."
— Kevin Nealon

"The time will come when men such as I will look upon the murder of animals as they now look on the murder of men."
— Leonardo da Vinci, Scientist and Artist

The animals on our plates

"So you are the people tearing down the Brazilian rainforest and breeding cattle."
– Prince Philip to McDonald's of Canada

"You're thinking I'm one of those wise-ass California vegetarians who is going to tell you that eating a few strips of bacon is bad for your health. I'm not. I say its a free country and you should be able to kill yourself at any rate you choose, as long as your cold dead body is not blocking my driveway."
– Scott Adams, Author of Dilbert

"Until we have the courage to recognize cruelty for what it is – whether its victim is human or animal – we cannot expect things to be much better in this world. We cannot have peace among men whose hearts delight in killing any living creature. By every act that glorifies or even tolerates such moronic delight in killing we set back the progress of humanity."
– Rachel Carson, Author and Scientist

"If you knew how meat was made, you'd probably lose your lunch."
– k.d. lang, Musician

"Animals are my friends… and I don't eat my friends."
– George Bernard Shaw, Playwright, Spokesman and Philosopher

The Fast Food Craze

"Aside from the health, environmental and animal rights reasons to be vegetarian, as an artist, I also consider it a matter of aesthetics. To me, our world is a more beautiful place if it is life affirmative. Nature has given us such a wonderful abundance of plant food, and we don't have to destroy other life to feed ourselves. As a vegan, I also feel that my sustenance is not at the cost of others—as a result of making more arable land available for food for people rather than feed for livestock. To me, the greatest way I can use my art is to visualize a beautiful, peaceful, humane planet, and my vegan lifestyle is a big part of that."
– Peter Max

In the U.S. alone, 500,000 animals are killed for meat every hour.

Every time I think about these animals and read quotes by people who are compassionate about them it brings me literally to tears. I want so badly to be able to help them, to free them. To explain to their little souls how sorry I am that all of this is happening to them. I feel so overwhelmed at the injustice of it all and so small and insignificant in such a huge world. All I can hope is that this reaches you and you understand, and your neighbor and family understand and you help me spread the message, because, as God is our witness, these animals need *help*.

Being a vegetarian has health benefits, however it has even better benefits if you happen to care about the animals on our planet. I have researched this subject for years, and that research compelled me without reserve to become a complete vegetarian. My research centered on animals that are raised for food. Do you know that there are very few laws restricting the cruel treatment of animals raised for food? Somehow, the almighty dollar has raised its ugly head again, this time in the agribusiness. The players seem to have lost all human compassion and caring and have decided that what they are dealing with is just meat for money. They don't want to see the sad faces or the living creature inside trying to somehow exist in these horrible conditions. Death would be so much more of a comfort. It is so sad because the animals in this environment are such wonderful creatures, left to their own devices. Here are some examples . . .

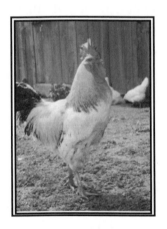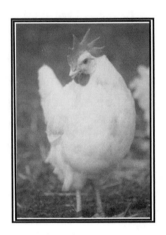

A beautiful rooster . . . a healthy hen!

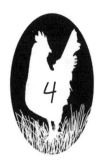

Chickens

The mother hen, how could she have known?

Chicken: The word is often used as a term for coward, but the opposite is true about these creatures. Roosters are known for their pride, ferocity and assertion of their power. The hens are not the meek creatures we have been taught they are. They can be fierce in defending their little ones, even against the most predatory animals. We have been conditioned to think these creatures are stupid. If an animal does something we call it instinct, if we as humans do something, we call it intelligence. We have a very self-serving way of measuring intelligence. The more I have learned about chickens, the more I realize what intelligent, caring, loving creatures they really are.

One naturalist gave a chicken hen some duck eggs just to see what would happen. Oddly, the chicken took to the job like a champ and did her motherly thing, lying on the eggs. The eggs hatched and the mother hen still didn't care that they weren't chickens, she took to them like her own. The little ducks were large, and didn't look like chickens. But this hen realized what these ducks needed, and wandered down by the creek. She jumped on a log, crossing the creek, and directed the little ducklings into the water, knowing that this is what they wanted and needed.

How could she have known? What form of intelligence was she using? It is a mystery how this chicken hen knew what these babies needed, but she did. We may not have much personal experience with chickens anymore, so we probably don't know what wonderful mothers they really are! The Romans had so much respect for the mothering nature of the chicken hen, they frequently used the term "son of a hen," to mean a well-cared for man.

Chickens like to explore their surroundings in a variety of ways using their sensitive beaks to probe the soil in search of food. The beak is also used for grooming and dust bathing. They also explore their environment and search for food by scratching with their feet. Chickens senses are acute—they have excellent vision, seeing color ranges similar to humans. A study showed that the music of choice for some chickens is Vivaldi's *The Four Seasons*—the "Spring" section caused the birds to playfully run, jump, and chase one another. Chickens also enjoy playing with toys. In a loving environment they have been known to bond with humans and other pets and show love, actually cooing to show their appreciation.

Chickens are inquisitive and interesting animals and are thought to be as intelligent as mammals like cats and dogs and even primates. When in natural surroundings, not on factory farms, they form friendships and social hierarchies, recognize one another, love their young, and enjoy a full life, dust-bathing, making nests, roosting in trees, and more.

Up until a few years ago, few scientists had spent any time learning about chickens' intelligence, but people who run farmed animal sanctuaries have had plenty to say about the subtleties of the chicken world. It may seem odd, since we don't know chickens very well, but it's true that some chickens like classic rock, while others like classical music; some chickens enjoy human company, while others are standoffish, shy, or even a bit aggressive. Just like dogs, cats, and humans, each chicken is an individual with a distinct personality. Now, scientists are beginning to learn a bit more about chickens, and here's what a few of them have to say:

- Chickens are as smart as mammals, including some primates, according to animal behaviorist Dr. Chris Evans, who runs the animal behavior lab at Macquarie University in Australia and lectures on his work with chickens. He explains that, for example, chickens are able to understand that recently hidden objects still exist, which is actually beyond the capacity of small children. Discussing chickens' various capacities, he says, "As a trick at conferences I sometimes list these attributes, without mentioning chickens, and people think I'm talking about monkeys."

- Dr. Joy Mench, professor and director of the Center for Animal Welfare at the University of California at Davis explains, "Chickens show sophisticated social behavior. ... That's what a pecking order is all about. They can recognize more than a hundred other chickens and remember them. They have more than thirty types of vocalizations."

- In her book *The Development of Brain and Behaviour in the Chicken,* Dr. Lesley Rogers, a professor of neuroscience and animal behavior, concludes that chickens have cognitive capabilities equivalent to mammals.

- Dr. Christine Nicol of the University of Bristol explains, "Chickens have shown us they can do things people didn't think they could do. There are hidden depths to chickens, definitely."

A Few Examples of Chicken Capabilities

- The video *Let's Ask the Animals,* produced by the Association for the Study of Animal Behaviour in the United Kingdom, shows chickens learning which bowls contain food by watching television, learning to peck a button three times in order to obtain food, and learning how to navigate a complex obstacle course in order to get to a nesting box.

- In 2002, the PBS documentary *The Natural History of the Chicken* revealed that "chickens love to watch television and have vision similar to humans. They also seem to enjoy all forms of music, especially classical."

- Chickens are able to learn by watching the mistakes of others and are very adept at teaching and learning.

- Chickens also can learn to use switches and levers to change the temperature in their surroundings and to open doors to feeding areas.

- Chickens have more than thirty distinct cries to communicate to one another, including separate alarm calls depending on whether a predator is traveling by land or sea.

- A mother hen will turn her eggs as many as five times an hour and cluck to her unborn chicks, who will chirp back to her and to one another from within their shells!

- Chickens navigate by the sun.

- A hen will often go without food and water, if necessary, just to have a private nest in which to lay her eggs.

- Like us, chickens form strong family ties and mourn when they lose a loved one.

Source: PETA website, www.peta.org/feat/hiddenlives/

With Love for Fryer Tuck

by Jan Whalen

The sun beats down on my back so warm and soft, just like the gentle rooster I am holding in my arms. We swing slowly back and forth in the big yard swing. Fryer Tuck's eyes are closed, he rests his head gently on my shoulder, as he has done before, only this time is special in a different way. It is a time for dreaming and recalling the good life he has had here with the Biddy Bums, my affectionate name for my pet chickens. You see, I run an orphanage for stray and abused poultry and have built for them a small Victorian house in my backyard called the Cob Web Cottage, which is part of my Feather Bed and Breakfast for tourists.

Sixteen months ago, I got a call from some people who had visited a chicken slaughterhouse to survey the carnage, when to their surprise seven young birds were discovered hiding under the machinery. The rest is history. I took in the whole dung-covered, crippled, and sick lot, whom we called The Fryers Club including Fryer Tuck, Rob Hen Hood, Maid Mary Hen, and Little John!

Fryer Tuck and I have seen a lot since then. Together we watched his little band die, one by one, of diseases caused by the demand for meat. To most people who come here, that's all chickens are, until they get to know Fryer Tuck, and hear his story, and see how much I love him.

I hug him tighter. His eyes are closed, and I remember

Chickens—The mother hen, how could she have known?

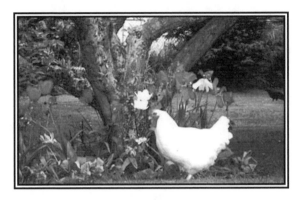

Fryer Tuck

the time that he went to my friend Lois's home as an honored birthday guest and impressed everyone with his nice house manners. I think of the many times that he made his way into the hearts of children just by being himself, and letting them pet him, while I told the story of his great escape. He's been quite an ambassador for animal rights.

I stroke him once more, and my tears fall, not so much for him as for me. For you see, the lovable big rooster who lies in my arms with his head on my shoulder died in his sleep during the night. He was the last member of the Fryer's Club. When I tucked him in, I remember hugging him and telling him how much I loved him. I told him, "You know honey, Mom wouldn't be here at midnight checking on you and caring for you if she didn't love you so much."

Little children will ask about him, and I'll tell them the truth, that he is in heaven. They may cry too, but it will be for his good fortune, and we will work together so that one day all the other chickens and factory farm animals will have as good a life as Fryer Tuck had, because all the people who say they love animals will have quit eating them.

Sitting here dreaming of that day, I love you, Fryer Tuck, and promise that the Fryers Club will never be forgotten.

Rhoda

by Karen Davis, Ph.D., founder United Poultry Concerns

I found Rhoda, a Rhode Island Red hen, at a local animal shelter. Her feathers were so matted she seemed to have been living inside a box or crate for some time, and she had an offensive discharge suggesting a prolonged ovary or kidney infection. The volunteer shelter staff had balked at having to feed her because she was "just a chicken."

From the beginning, Rhoda was a gentle and affectionate hen who liked being petted and held. The morning after bringing her home I placed her outside on the grass in the sun. So abruptly did she collapse on her side, close her eyes, and stretch out her wing in a long arc of feathers across the ground that I thought she had died. I lay down beside her. Still, she was breathing, so I let her alone, and for a long time, twenty minutes or more, she never moved so much as an eyelid, and then only to shift herself to allow the other side of her body to take in all the warm sunshine.

Chickens—The mother hen, how could she have known?

Rhoda shared our house where she spent most of her days soaking up the spots of sunbeam that appeared on the floor. The kitchen doorstep was her favorite sunny place. Several times I carried her in my arms down our little pathway out back to visit with Muffie and Fluffie and Henry, our other three chickens who were then living in an old hen house with a fenced-in tomato garden for a yard. Henry was a young, heavy rooster who had fallen off the truck on the way to the slaughterhouse the summer before. He was very attracted to Rhoda, I could tell. Whenever we appeared, he'd plot eagerly over to the fence and stand there regarding her, then follow us on the inside of the fence as we started to go.

One day after Rhoda had been with us a few weeks, she disappeared from the house. My husband and I searched everywhere. Finally, we went down the little path looking for her. Sure enough, there was Rhoda, conversing with Henry through the fence. She seemed to be getting better under the antibiotics, we felt. Touchingly, after a few minutes, she walked behind us back to the house, and for the first and last time, proceeded to give herself a vigorous dust bath under the big bush at the foot of the kitchen step. It was late afternoon. From this time on, for reasons unclear, Rhoda grew steadily weaker, and within a few days she was dead. We buried her beneath the trees along-side the little pathway not far from where our Henry has since been laid in the ground as well.

Chickens in Factory Farms

Now let's talk about what these creatures endure on a daily basis, for their entire lives.

In egg farms, the male chickens aren't needed so what happens to them? As soon as they poke there little precious heads out of their shells, they are swooped up and thrown into a large plastic trash bag to suffocate among their brothers. And their lives are actually better than the ones who survive.

With the growing number of humans trying to limit their intake of red meat, the poultry industries are booming. Record numbers of chickens and turkeys are being raised and killed for meat in the U.S. every year. Nearly 10 billion chickens and 0.5 billion turkeys are hatched in one year. Chickens are social and need to have some sort of pecking order to survive. Their brains are not only trained for finding food and water, there is a lot more that goes on in their instinctive lives.

In factory farms these chickens have no natural sunlight, and have lost the opportunity to live their lives as nature intended. Because of this, they are literally driven insane. They peck at each other, scream, and sometimes are driven so insane, they resort to cannibalism. Chickens who are over-crowded and who are driven insane by this, tend to panic and jump on top of one another, killing the chickens below by smothering them. The farmers have also remedied this situation. They have decided that if they crowded the birds even more tightly, they would not be able to jump on top of each other and kill more profits. They are living in such crowded circumstances that just getting to the scientific food fed them and the water, is nearly impossible. Some of the weaker birds never make it to the food and water and end up dying of starvation and dehydration.

The people who run these factory farms have remedied the pecking situation too! It's called de-beaking. This procedure is probably the most painful thing that can be done to a chicken. Between the horn and the bone is a thin layer of highly sensitive soft tissue resembling the quick of the human nail. The hot knife used in de-beaking cuts through this complex of horn and sensitive tissue, causing *severe* pain. This is done without any anesthesia or painkillers, they cut off the most sensitive part of the chickens, their beaks, so that when they do go insane and start pecking and screaming, they won't do much damage to the others. It's all about profits you know.

Today's broiler chicken (meat) have been genetically altered to grow twice as fast and twice as large as their ancestors. In this process, hundreds of millions of chickens die every year before even reaching slaughter. They grow so fast that the heart and lungs are not developed and the results are congestive heart failure and tremendous death losses. They also experience crippling leg disorders due to abnormally heavy bodies. Confined in unsanitary, disease-ridden factory farms, the birds also succumb to heat prostration, infectious diseases, and cancer.

Chickens and turkeys are taken to the slaughterhouse in crates stacked on the backs of open trucks. When they arrive from their factory farm life (hell), they are either pulled from their crates or dumped onto a conveyor belt. Some miss the belt and die an even more grim death. Some die from being crushed by machinery or others may die of starvation or exposure days, or even weeks later. Birds inside the slaughterhouse suffer an equally gruesome fate. They are fully conscious and hung by their feet by metal shackles on a moving rail. Chickens are excluded from the federal Human Slaughter Act, which requires stunning prior to slaughter, many are placed in electrified water baths to immobilize them to hurry assembly line killing. This procedure is even crueler because of concerns that too much electricity would damage the carcass, so they usually remain conscious and are still capable of feeling pain and fear. After the shackled birds pass through the stunning tank, their throats are slashed, usually by a mechanical blade. Inevitably the blade misses some birds, who may still be struggling and moving. The next thing that happens is the scalding tank. The ones that weren't fortunate enough to have the blade hit them are literally scalded alive. This occurs so often that the industry has a term for them. They call them "redskins."

Take the Chickens and Run!
How 10 battery-caged hens came to live at UPC
by Jim Sicard

The first door was locked. So was the second. And the third. Damn! Months earlier, they'd been tipped off about a hen factory in Maryland. A fireman who went there to put out a fire told UPC (United Poultry Concerns) he'd never seen anything like it—that was the last egg he'd ever eat. Dressed in black and armed with a video camera, they made the two-hour trip. In the back of the truck were blankets, pillowcases, a camcorder, camera, night-vision goggles, gloves, surgical masks, a flashlight, and a pry bar.

At one o'clock a.m., they made their journey across the field to the compound. Ten minutes and two fences later, they stood before five buildings. A few trucks and trailers were scattered about.

The fifth door opened. They went in. Inside, the buildings were attached to one another by a hall through which the eggs went by a conveyer belt to a sixth building where they were crated and loaded on trucks. What they experienced was so horrible one couldn't imagine it. No wonder the workers wore full face ventilators. The air was vile with ammonia, 90 degrees, dusty, moist, and sickening.

They went on with their plan. First they filmed the place. Rows of cages the size of a doormat to the floor, each one stuffed with de-beaked hens with spindly long claws and limp, lifeless wattles. They walked slowly down the aisles filming these poor souls. Occasionally a hen started when the camera went off; otherwise they barely moved.

Stage two, the rescue. They decided to take ten hens, but which ones? In the end it was random. They selected a bank of cages and pulled out the pillowcases. They slid open the gate on top of a cage. It was narrower than the hens' bodies. It took them longer to carefully pull out one terrified hen clinging to the wire than it would have taken the catchers to empty several cages. They put ten hens in three pillowcases and took off. Ten minutes after running and stumbling across the field in the dark, they gently opened the pillowcases into the back of the truck.

The hens lay still the entire ride back. Maybe they would die but at least they were out of there. They were weak, but as time showed, tough. A couple of hours later, they were at United Poultry Concerns. Free at last!

Three months later the change in these hens is amazing. In March they were ravaged, scraggly bodies with doughy combs and murky eyes. Now they run around the yard on their strong little legs with snowy feathers, red combs, bright eyes, and claws almost normal. Sweet Pea, Portia, Pearl, and Pia perch together every night. What's especially wonderful is to walk outside and see two or three of these beautiful hens resting quietly in the branches of a tree.

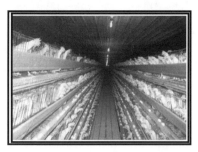

Welcome to chicken hell

Chickens—The mother hen, how could she have known?

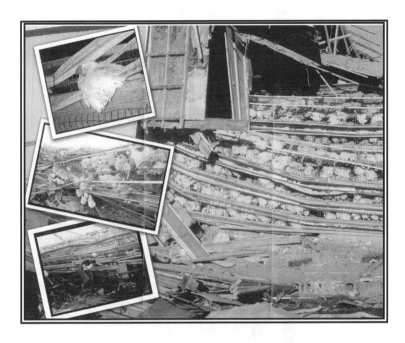

The "wonderful" agribusiness

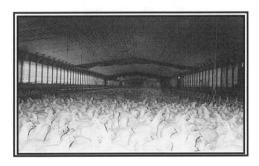

Void of natural sunlight and dirt . . .

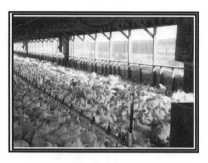

*Living on top of one another,
for lack of space*

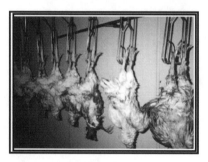

*Alive . . .
and ready for slaughter!*

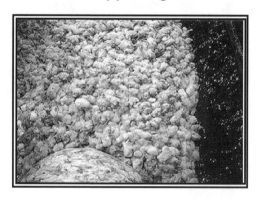

*Here is what happens to the male chicks
at egg factories.*

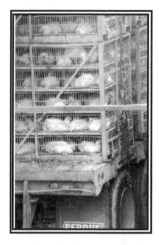

*On their way to a
better life—death*

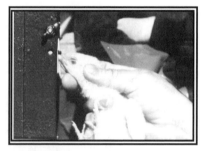

*This little chick has done
nothing to deserve this horrible
pain*

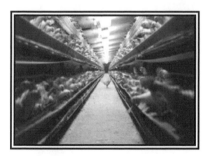

*False lights to trick the hens
into laying more eggs*

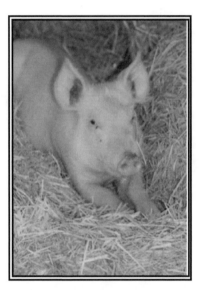

A healthy piglet,
undamaged by factory life

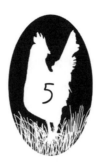

5

Pigs
Smart enough to be saving lives?

Pigs are intelligent beings. Dogs look up to us, cats look down on us, pigs treat us as equals. Pigs are loyal by nature and often form close friendships with one another. Physical contact is very important to them. Pigs enjoy close contact with humans and form very strong bonds with humans as well. They like being scratched behind the ears and shoulders, grunting contentedly, and will happily roll over for belly rubs. They are very vocal. They use over twenty identified vocalizations to constantly communicate with one another. Males and females have a song they use when courting, and pigs also enjoy music. Newborn piglets learn to come to their mother's voice, and the mother pig "sings" to her young as they nurse. Pigs are very clean animals and discriminating eaters. They carefully keep their sleeping area clean and will designate a spot as far from this area as possible for waste. Unable to sweat, they bathe in mud to cool themselves and to protect their skin from insects and sun. They prefer water to mud, however, and are good swimmers.

Pigs are intelligent and like puppies, piglets will learn their names and come when called. They are loyal companions and have saved people from harm.

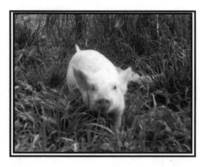

Pigs—Smart enough to be saving lives?

Priscilla, a 2-month-old piglet, saves a young boy from drowning

Adapted from Real Animal Heroes *by Paul Drew*

One hot July day in 1984, Carol Burk and her 11-year-old son, Anthony, went swimming in Texas' Lake Somerville. They were joined by Priscilla, a twentytwo-pound, two-month-old piglet they had raised. Priscilla loved the water and was a great swimmer, but Anthony, a mentally handicapped child, was not.

For hours, Anthony, his mother, and Priscilla played hide-and-seek in the shallow waters. Finally, Anthony tired and his mom turned to get ready to leave. When she turned back, Anthony was far out in the water, struggling. She started swimming toward him, and so did Priscilla. Despite being very tired from swimming all day, the little pig reached Anthony first. He grabbed for her halter and leash. In his panic he pulled too hard and went under, this time taking Priscilla with him!

Now both Anthony and Priscilla were drowning and he weighed almost four times more than she did. Priscilla struggled to get to the surface of the water. Finally, with enormous effort, she succeeded. With Anthony clinging to her small body, Priscilla swam back to shore.

Priscilla, like all pigs, has a very long memory. Years after the rescue, she still became upset whenever she saw young children playing near the water. For her heroism, Priscilla was honored with a "Priscilla the Pig" day in Houston, Texas.

Another great pig story came to me from a friend who was an eyewitness to this event. This is about a pot-bellied pig that lived in a little wood frame house with his owner, a woman named Jean. Jean was sixty-eight-years old and had no other companion than Rudy, whom she had raised from a piglet. Rudy and Jean were the best of friends, they watched TV together and had their meals together. Rudy was like a child to Jean.

One day, Jean had a heart attack and fell down and could not get up. Rudy did not know what to do, but he knew Jean was in trouble. He ran out the door to the *middle of the street and lay down, waiting for another human to come by and help Jean. He did this continually for hours, running back in the house to check on Jean, then running back out and lying down in the street. Finally someone stopped. Rudy actually figured out how to let the person in the car know to follow him into the house. He saved Jean that day. It took him awhile, but if it hadn't been for him, she would have died on that floor. Smart Pig!*

Pigs in Factory Farms

While driving from Los Angeles to Chicago, Saverio Truglia stopped at a truck stop in southern Utah to make a sandwich for lunch. "Suddenly," he said, "the air became laden with the smells of live hogs." He tried to ignore the pungent odors blowing toward him. "What I couldn't ignore," he said, "was the heated life-and-death struggle occurring inside the semi's perforated steel shell. Snouts and mouths jutted through air holes while human-looking eyes stared to the outside." Truglia went over to the trailer and peered inside. He saw "a sea of enormous pink hogs, all struggling for space in the cramped container. Those pigs that somehow got lifted up by the dense crowd were riding the others, with front hooves gouging the bloody backs of those who managed to keep all fours on the ground. This caused considerable panic and certainly pain in the surrounding animals." Knowing how intelligent pigs are, Truglio spoke to the pigs at the Utah truck stop. His voice momentarily calmed them, long enough for him to shoot a roll of film. Then the driver pulled the semi away, headed for the slaughterhouse.

Source: PETA website, www.Peta.org/literature

The corporate hog factories have taken over the traditional hog farms and pigs raised for food are being treated as lifeless tools of production, rather than as living, feeling animals.

Approximately 100 million pigs are raised and slaughtered in the U.S. every year. As babies, they are subjected to painful mutilations without anesthesia or pain relievers. Their tails are cut off to minimize tail biting, something that happens when these highly intelligent animals are kept in deprived factory farm conditions. In addition, notches are taken out of the piglet's ears for identification. By two to three weeks of age, 15% of the piglets have died. Those who do, are taken away from their mothers and crowded into pens with metal bars and concrete floors. A headline from *National Hog Farmer* magazine says "Crowding Pigs Pays . . . " and this is shown by the intense over-crowding in every stage of a pigs confinement system. Pigs live this way, packed into giant, warehouse-like sheds, until they reach a slaughter weight of 250 pounds at six months old.

The air in hog factories is laden with dust, dander and noxious gases, which are produced as the animals' urine and feces builds up inside the sheds. For pigs, which spend their entire lives in these conditions, respiratory disease is rampant. Many other diseases are reported that are horribly painful and inhumane. Modern breeding sows are treated like piglet-making machines . . . living a continuous cycle of breeding and birth. Each sow has more than twenty piglets a year. When pregnant, the sows are confined in gestation crates—small metal pens just two feet wide to prevent them from turning around or even lying down comfortably. At the end of their four-month pregnancies, they are transferred to similar cramped crates to give birth. With barely enough room to stand up and lie down, and no bedding to speak of, many suffer from sores on their shoulders and knees. When asked about this, one pork industry representative wrote ". . . straw is very expensive and there certainly would not be a supply of straw in the country to supply all of the birthing pens in the U.S."

The psychological damage this does to pigs is unbelievable. After the sows give birth and nurse their young for two to three weeks, the piglets are taken away to be fattened and the sows are re-impregnated.

In addition to overcrowded housing, sows and pigs also endure extreme crowding in transportation to slaughter, resulting in rampant suffering and deaths.

Prior to being hung upside down by their back legs and bled to death at the slaughterhouse, pigs are supposed to be "stunned" and rendered unconscious, in accordance with the federal Humane Slaughter Act. However, stunning at slaughterhouses is terribly inexact, and often conscious animals are hung upside down, kicking and struggling, while a slaughterhouse worker tries to "stick" them in the neck with a knife. If the worker is unsuccessful, the pig will be carried (still kicking and struggling) to the next station . . . the scalding tank . . . where he/she will be boiled, alive and fully conscious.

On October 1, en route from a North Carolina factory farm to a Pennsylvania slaughterhouse, nearly two hundred five-month-old pigs, crammed onto a triple-deck transport trailer, were abandoned by their driver in northeast D.C. Found by D.C.

Animal Control, the vehicle was towed to Poplar Spring Animal Sanctuary in Poolesville, Maryland. Responding to the urgent situation, local animal activists rushed to Poplar Spring to help unload the animals into a four-acre pasture at the sanctuary.

Victims of modern day factory farming, the pigs, who had never touched dirt before, were covered in urine and feces and had burn marks from electric prodding all over their bodies. Upon arriving at the sanctuary, several were found dead on the truck, a common result of overcrowding. Walking over the dead bodies of pigs who had been stomped to death or died from stress seizures, the survivors stumbled awkwardly off the truck and into the pasture.

Due to intense confinement, most were unable to walk without severe leg cramping and pain. For several consecutive days, activists worked around the clock to feed, clean, and provide fresh water for the animals. Needless to say, after experiencing the torture of factory farm existence, the pigs didn't know how to react to kind treatment.

When the factory farmer learned of the botched transport, he demanded that his "property" be returned. A press release was sent out and nearly every media outlet in D.C. arrived at Poplar Spring on October 2, coincidentally World Farm Animals Day (Gandhi's birthday). Exposing the gross abuse suffered by the pigs, the media closely documented the showdown between animal activists and the pork industry.

The story appeared on the front page of the Washington Post's Metro section and was the feature story of almost every major news station that evening.

To make a long story short, by October 3, the veterinary, food, and housing bill incurred during the pigs' stay had risen above their financial worth ($12,000). Hence, in lieu of paying the bill, the factory farmer agreed to simply sign over custody of all 167 survivors to Poplar Spring Animal Sanctuary. A victorious news release was sent out, and the story was once again featured on every major news station that evening, some even doing live segments from the sanctuary. Several radio stations covered the story as well.

Today, the pigs are living in peace and safety at various animal sanctuaries along the East Coast. Never again will they be in danger of losing their lives to the profit-over-ethics mentality inherent to the human supremacist attitude.

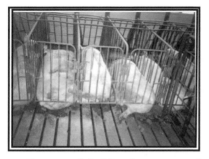
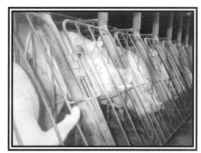

Imagine life like this . . . not being able to turn around, EVER

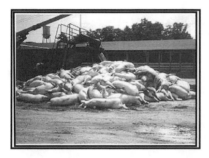
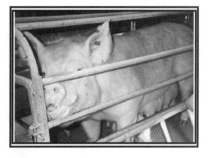

These pigs were just too sick; the top ones are probably still alive.

Begging for attention or someone to save them.

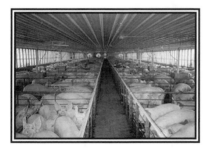
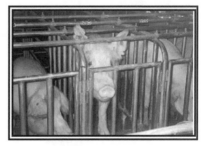

Fighting for a small place to call their own.

Dying for attention

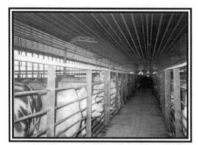

Cramped beyond belief

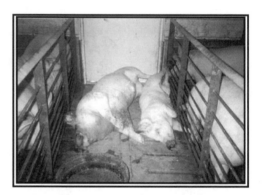

Sick and unable to get up

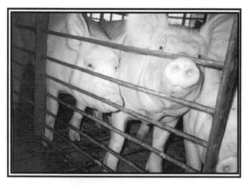

Poor, poor babies

Pigs: Smart enough to be saving lives?

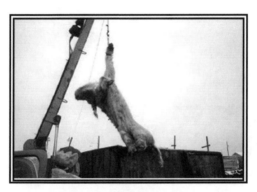

Treated just like meat . . .

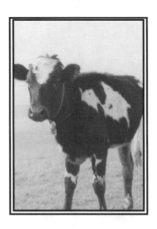

Sweet, gentle, and kind

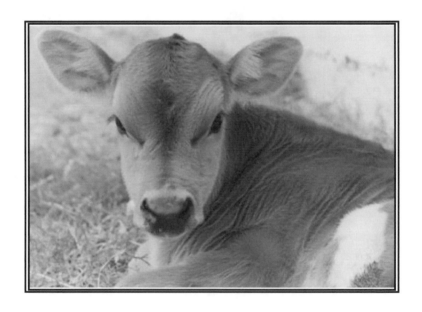

A happy calf, meant to live life as God intended.

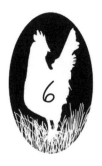

Cows
Sweet, gentle, and kind

Cows have a special kind of intelligence and sensitivity. But, because they are such patient and gentle souls who rarely hurry or make a fuss about things, we tend to think they are dumb, and don't recognize their unique presence. Rooted deeply in the rhythms of the earth, they move through life with a peacefulness that is not easy to disturb. They are not troubled by much of what bothers us, and when they are alarmed, usually by things we cannot see, they are still slow to panic, and rarely overreact. Few of us today, have much opportunity to experience for ourselves what kind of creatures cattle are. A naturalist who knew cows well, W. H. Hudson, spoke movingly of ". . . the gentle, large-brained, social cow, that caresses our hands and faces with her rough blue tongue, and is more like a man's sister than any other non-human being—the majestic, beautiful creature with the Juno eyes . . ."

Cows exhibit affection and loyalty to humans. Mother cows share "babysitting" duties with one or two cows watching all the calves while the other mother cows graze. As calves grow up together and have calves of their own, their calves may also befriend each other.

The Story of Queenie

She made a daring dash from a New York City slaughterhouse in Queens . . . and won the hearts of thousands of people who joined her quest for freedom.

We're talking, of course, about "Queenie," a young cow who was slated for slaughter at Astoria Live Poultry, a meat market that keeps live animals and allows customers to choose the animals they want butchered. After hearing the screams of other animals, Queenie made her own choice— a choice any animal would make in the same situation if given a chance. After escaping from the slaughterhouse, Queenie ran several blocks through the streets of New York City, surprising motorists and passers-by. Though she avoided capture at first, the five-hundred-pound cow was finally caught after a wild chase with NYPD cars, local authorities, and a tranquilizer gun.

Director Gene Bauston tells reporter about Queenie's heroic escape to freedom:

Queenie's freedom dash was quickly picked up by the media—and her story spread throughout the country. Queenie's courageous escape was featured on national television, and millions of viewers saw a frightened cow running from the slaughterhouse, clearly aware of the fate that had awaited her.

Hundreds of calls poured into The Center for Animal Care and Control and Astoria Live Poultry, urging both the agency and the slaughterhouse owner to release the animal to a sanctuary where she could live out the remainder of her life.

Alerted to the cow's plight by Farm Sanctuary members, we immediately contacted the animal control agency and offered to provide Queenie a safe, loving, permanent home. For several hours, it was unclear if the agency would obtain custody of the cow, but public sentiment and pressure paid off—and the slaughterhouse owner agreed to give the cow to the city. In statements to newspapers, Aladdin El-sayed, owner of Astoria Live Poultry, which is a halal slaughterhouse stated, "God was willing to give it a new life, so why wouldn't I?" *(Newsday)*.

El-sayed also stated he had paid $500 for the cow, and had been fined $1,000 for causing an "animal nuisance." The Health Department may fine him an additional $2,000. El-sayed claimed he "lost a lot of money," but that it didn't matter because, in his own words, "There is something with this cow." *(Daily News)*

After receiving the word on Friday afternoon that Queenie would be given to Farm Sanctuary, our animal transport vehicle was rolling to New York City by Friday night. We picked up Queenie from the JFK Airport where she was being held, and drove her directly to our New York shelter. Queenie jumped off the trailer amid cheers from the sanctuary staff . . . and loud "welcome" moo's from the shelter cows.

That's Some Cow

Queenie has put a face on vegetarianism. With news stories on the major television networks, Associated Press, and articles in *The New York Times, New York Daily News,* and dozens of other newspapers, millions of people have learned that farm animals have feelings too.

Queenie's quest has also launched a neighborhood effort to close the slaughterhouse. Like Queenie seizing her moment for freedom, residents have seized the news attention to draw attention to their demand to close the meat market. Among their concerns reported in the *New York Post,* residents stated, "This is a market that we don't believe is treating anything humanely, and we want to see it closed for that reason alone . . . Through the night, you can hear the screaming of the animals. I don't know what they are doing to them."

Queenie knew . . . and now the rest of the world knows, too.

Cows in Factory Farms

"At stockyards, I have seen cows dragged with ropes because they are too sick or injured to walk. I watched a dairy cow with a broken pelvis being moved in a bulldozer. I have seen a number of cows unable to walk [transported] in the bucket of bulldozers. At a slaughterhouse, I saw a newborn calf separated from her mother and left to die. Baby male Holstein dairy calves barely able to walk were being auctioned off daily. I saw a cow unable to walk dumped outside on a pile of dead animals, where she . . . froze." — *Julie Derby, PETA slaughterhouse investigator*

Many beef cattle are born and live on the range, foraging and fending for themselves for months or even years. They are not adequately protected against inclement weather and may die of dehydration or freeze to death.

Accustomed to roaming unbothered and relaxed, range cattle are frightened and confused when humans come to round them up. Terrified animals are often injured, some so severely that they become "downed" (unable to walk or even stand). These downed animals suffer for days without receiving food, water, or veterinary care, and many die of neglect. Others are dragged, beaten, and pushed with tractors on their way to slaughter. Many cattle will experience more transportation and handling stress at stockyards and auctions, where they are pushed through a series of walkways and holding pens and sold to the highest bidder.

Ranchers still identify cattle the same way they have since pioneer days—with hot iron brands. Needless to say, this prac-tice is extremely traumatic and painful, and the animals bellow loudly as rancher's brands are burned into their skin. Beef cattle are also subjected to "waddling," another type of identification marking. This painful procedure entails cutting chunks out of the hide that hangs under the animals' necks. Waddling marks are supposed to be large enough so that ranchers can identify their cattle from a distance.

Most beef cattle spend the last few months of their lives at feed lots, crowded by the thousands into dusty, manure-laden holding pens. The air is thick with harmful bacteria and particulate matter, and the animals are at constant risk for respiratory disease. Feed lot cattle are routinely implanted with growth-promoting hormones, and they are fed unnaturally rich diets designed to fatten them up quickly and profitably. Because cattle are biologically suited to eat a grass-based, high fiber diet, their concentrated feed lot rations contribute to metabolic disorders.

Cattle may be transported several times during their lifetimes, and they may travel hundreds or even thousands of miles during a single trip. Long journeys are very stressful and contribute to disease and even death. The Drover's Journal reports, "Shipping fever costs livestock producers as much as $1 billion per year."

Young cattle are commonly taken to areas with cheap grazing land, to take advantage of this inexpensive feed source. Upon reaching maturity, they are trucked to a feedlot to be fattened and readied for slaughter. Eventually, all of them will end up at the slaughterhouse.

A standard beef slaughterhouse kills 250 cattle every hour. The high speed of the assembly line makes it increasingly difficult to provide animals with any resemblance of humane treatment. A *Meat & Poultry* article states:

> Good handling is extremely difficult if equipment is 'maxed out' all the time. It is impossible to have a good attitude toward cattle if employees have to constantly

overexert themselves, and thus transfer all that stress right down to the animal, just to keep up with the line.

Prior to being hung up by their back legs and bled to death, cattle are supposed to be rendered unconscious, as stipulated by the federal Humane Slaughter Act. This "stunning" is usually done by a mechanical blow to the head. However, the procedure is terribly faulty, and inadequate stunning is inevitable. As a result, conscious animals are often hung upside down, kicking and struggling, while a slaughterhouse worker makes another attempt to render them unconscious. Eventually the animals will be "stuck" in the throat with a knife, and blood will gush from their bodies, whether or not they are unconscious. This is detailed in an April 2001, *Washington Post* article, which describes typical slaughter plant conditions:

> The cattle were supposed to be dead before they got to Moreno. But too often there weren't.
>
> They blink. They make noises, he said softly. The head moves, the eyes are wide and looking around. Still Moreno would cut. On bad days, he says, dozens of animals reached his station clearly alive and conscious. Some would survive as far as the tail cutter, the belly ripper, the hide puller. They die, said Moreno, piece by piece . . .

"In plants all over the U.S. this happens on a daily basis," said Lester Friedlander, a veterinarian and formerly chief government inspector at a Pennsylvania hamburger plant. "I've seen it happen. And I've talked to other veterinarians. They feel it's out of control."

The U.S. Department of Agriculture oversees the treatment of animals in meat plants, but enforcement of the law varies dramatically. While a few plants have been forced to halt production for a few hours because of alleged animal cruelty, such sanctions are rare.

Reaction to the *Washington Post* article and others like it started a Congressional resolution reiterating the importance of the Humane Slaughter Act, but to date, there is little if any indication that the situation for animals in slaughterhouses has improved.

Dairy Cows

If you wouldn't drink milk from a dog or a giraffe, it's just as weird to drink milk from a cow! Human breast milk is designed for baby humans, giraffe milk is designed for baby giraffes, and cow's milk is designed for—yes—baby cows!

Cows produce milk for the same reason that humans do—to feed their newborns. Farmers must keep cows pregnant and delivering calves in order to get milk. Their calves are traumatically taken from their mothers just days after birth so that humans can drink the milk that nature intended for the infant calves. Female calves are slaughtered or raised to follow in their mothers' hoof prints. Male calves go to the veal industry to spend fourteen weeks chained in dark crates so tiny that they can't turn around in them. They see the light of day only on their way to slaughter.

On a typical dairy farm, cows stand on concrete, chained by the neck, in huge sheds and are milked by machines. To boost production, some farmers inject cows with synthetic growth hormones, which increase the cows' risk of developing mastitis, a painful condition that causes cows' udders to become so heavy that they sometimes drag on the ground.

Dr. John A. McDougall calls dairy foods "liquid meat" because they are as bad for you as the solid stuff. Loaded with fat and cholesterol, dairy products contribute to heart disease, cancer, stroke, diabetes, allergies, asthma, and even osteoporosis, the bone-weakening disease that the dairy industry pretends it prevents. It's easy to get plenty of calcium without milk—it's in tofu, all green leafy veggies, beans, nuts, and calcium-fortified orange juice and soy milk.

Regardless of where they live, all dairy cows must give birth in order to begin producing milk. Today, dairy cows are forced to birth a calf every year. Like human beings, cows have a nine-month gestation period, and so giving birth every twelve months is physically demanding. The cows are also artificially re-impregnated while they are still producing milk, so their bodies are still producing milk during seven months of their nine-month pregnancy. With genetic manipulation and intensive production technology, it is common for a cow to produce one hundred pounds of milk per day—ten times more than they would produce naturally. As a result, the cow's bodies are under constant stress and they are at risk for numerous health problems.

About half of the dairy cows suffer form of mastitis, a bacterial infection of their udders. This is such a common and costly ailment that a dairy industry group was formed specifically to combat the disease. Other diseases such as Bovine Leukemia Virus, Bovine Immunodeficiency Virus, and Johne's disease (the human manifestation is Crohn's disease) are also rampant on modern dairies, but they usually go unnoticed because they are either hard to detect or have a long incubation period. A cow eating a normal grass diet could not produce milk at these abnormal levels, so today's dairy cows must be given high- energy feeds. The unnaturally rich diet causes metabolic disorders including ketosis, which can be fatal, and laminitis, which causes lameness.

Another dairy industry disease caused by intensive milk production is "Milk Fever." This is caused by calcium deficiency, and it occurs when milk secretion depletes calcium faster than it can be replenished in the blood.

In a healthy environment, cows would live in excess of twenty-five years, but on modern dairies, they are slaughtered and made into ground beef after just three to four years. The abuse wreaked upon the bodies of dairy cows is so intense that the dairy industry also has a huge source of "downed animals."

Even though the dairy industry is familiar with the cow's health problems and suffering because of intensive milk production, it continues to subject cows to even worse abuses in the name of increased profit. Bovine Growth Hormone (BGH), a synthetic hormone, is now being injected into cows to get them to produce even more milk. Besides adversely affecting the cows' health, BGH also increases birth defects in their calves.

Calves born to dairy cows are separated from their mothers immediately after birth. The half that are born female are raised to replace older dairy cows in the milking herd. The male half are raised and slaughtered for meat. Most are killed for beef, but about one million are used for veal.

The veal industry was created a by-product of the dairy industry to take advantage of an abundant supply of unwanted male calves. Veal calves commonly live for eighteen to twenty weeks in wooden crates that are so small that they cannot turn around, stretch their legs, or even lie down comfortably. The calves are fed a liquid milk substitute, deficient in iron and fiber, which is designed to make the animals anemic, resulting in the light-colored flesh that is prized as veal. In addition to this high-priced veal, some calves are killed at just a few days old to be sold as low-grade "bob" veal for products like frozen TV dinners. These calves that are confined in crates exhibit abnormal coping behaviors associated with frustration. These include head tossing, head shaking, kicking, scratching, and chewing behavior. They also experience leg and joint disorders and an impaired ability to even walk.

Now let me ask you this: Are we prepared to actually eat these creatures that have suffered like this to feed us? How on earth can we consciously eat animals knowing that this is how their entire lives are spent? If reincarnation is a possibility, picture one of us coming back as a factory farmed animal. If we are all connected and share this earth the way God intended us to do, what are we to do about this gross abuse of lives, souls and common decency? Stop eating them. If every American stopped, even for one month, do you have any idea how many lives would be saved? It's in the billions. Let's try and save these animals, and give them back their God-given right.

Meet Your Meat

The video that all meat-eaters should watch and every vegetarian should own, *Meet Your Meat*, narrated by Alec Baldwin, covers each stage of life of animals raised for food.

More than 25 billion animals are killed for food every year in the United States. This video shows the lives and deaths of chickens, cows, and pigs and makes a poignant case for vegetarianism and humane legislation.

Pigs, cows, and chickens are individuals with feelings—they can feel love, happiness, loneliness, and fear, just as dogs, cats, and people do.

The purpose of factory farms is to produce the most meat, milk, and eggs using the least amount of space, time, and money. The animals suffer the consequences of these short-cuts. They are never allowed to do anything that is natural to them—they are never able to feel the grass beneath their feet, the sun on their faces, or fresh air.

They endure mutilation—chicks have their beaks burned off, cows and pigs are castrated without anesthesia, cows are dehorned and branded, and the list goes on—all without any painkillers. Some animals, such as veal calves, are kept in lonely isolation, while others, such as chickens, are crowded so closely together that they can barely move. Factory farmers restrict animals' movement, not only to save space, but also so that all their energy goes toward producing flesh, eggs, or milk for human consumption. They spend their lives confined to concrete stalls and metal cages, terrified and suffering in such unnatural conditions.

Their fear and pain end only after they have been driven, without food or water and often in extreme weather, to the mechanized murder of today's slaughterhouse, where millions each year are skinned and dismembered while still conscious.

Another must-see (and share) video is *Peaceable Kingdom,* by Farm Sanctuary. You can order right from the Farm Sanctuary website at www.farmsanctuary.org.

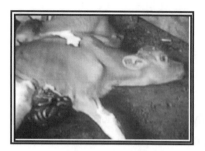

Due to the horrible factory conditions, this baby cow is too ill to stand.

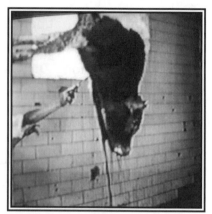

A cow, ready for slaughter. Her eyes are wide open; my God, what terror this poor animal must be feeling.

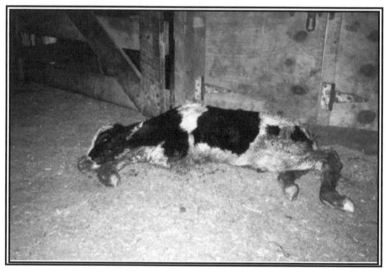

Another calf, too weak to stand

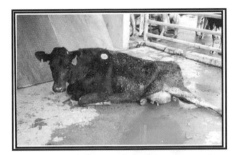

Another sick baby cow

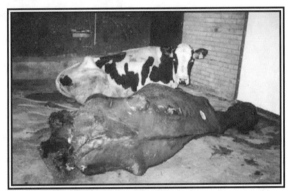

*The cruel treatment shows on the cow in the
foreground; the poor creature is all cut up*

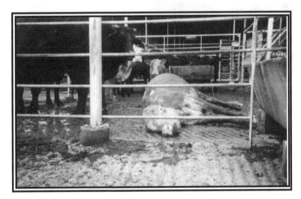

Sickness is rampant . . .

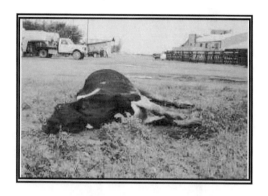

This cow was abandoned and left to die alone in a field, too sick to move.

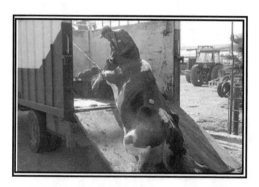

Imagine the terror this cow is feeling right at the moment this photo was taken . . .

7

What are we to do?

My suggestion to the problem of course is to stop eating animals and stop supporting the cruelty involved in putting animals in our food chain. Walking this earth with dead animals in our stomachs just seems very barbaric. Animals have suffered in unbelievable pain so that the super-markets and fast-food stores can put them in pretty packages to feed us. In my research, I have learned that it is not healthy, nor moral, to eat animals. These animals have as much a right to enjoy their lives as humans do. What gave humans the right to be the deciding factor in what happens in the lives of the animals? What happened to THEIR rights? What is this supremist attitude that has invaded the human race to say that it is okay to kill another living thing in order to feed ourselves, when God has given us so much on this earth to eat, without harming or killing?

Vegetarianism

The word "vegetarian" was coined by the vegetarian society of the United Kingdom in about 1847. The word does not come from vegetable as is generally assumed: it is the derivation of the Latin word *vegetarian* which means to enliven (or rejuvenate).

The practice of vegetarianism goes very far back in history. Many known philosophers & religious teachers urged their followers to avoid the flesh diet. Brahminism, Jainism, Zoroastrianism & Buddhism acknowledged the sacredness of life & the need to live without causing suffering; so did the early Christians.

Vegetarianism is thus a system based on scientific principles and has proved adequate for the best nutrition free from poisons and bacteria of diseased animals. It is the best diet for optimum physical, mental and spiritual development.

I was given meat on my plate as a youngster, and although I tried to slip it under the table for my dog to eat, my father was pretty stern about us kids getting our meat. There were times I was forced to eat it and it actually gagged me. I wish I would have been given a choice at that early age. My body knew that meat didn't belong in there. Since becoming a vegetarian, I am repulsed by the unsavory smells of cooked animals. When I walk into a Seven-11, for instance, the smell from the hot dogs nearly makes me sick. My point is that your body adjusts to a diet without animal products and it doesn't take long. You will not be able to tolerate meat products any longer. Your body will love you for it and you will be saving lives.

"Why become a vegetarian?"

This question was asked some visitors to International Vegetarian Union (IVU) website (www.ivu.org), and here were some pretty extraordinary answers:

If you have the chance to save one life—or to save thousands of lives—wouldn't you? Cutting animal products out of your life is a fairly simple thing you can do, with far reaching effects. The human animals are supposedly so evolved, with so many great gifts . . . shouldn't we use our gift of compassion to save other animals?
-Lise

To save yourself from the guilt of knowing that some animal died for you. Isn't that enough?? But for those skeptics, it's also a healthy habit.
-Lauren

To teach our children the sanctity of life and the true value of every living being, and to promote peace in them.
-Michelle

The single most effective thing you can do to help the most animals today, is to not eat them. Modern agriculture is a business, in it for the profit. Their concern is with doing things in the easiest and cheapest way, with little or no concern for the animals or their living souls.

ONE vegetarian will save the lives of 93 ANIMALS per year!

Vegetarian Studies:

After the Second World War, scientists began compiling data regarding the diets and health of all the populations in the world. One fact that came up repeatedly was that there was strong evidence between heavy flesh-eating people and a short life expectancy. The Eskimos, Laplanders, Greenlanders, and Russian Kurgi tribes stood out as the highest meat-eating populations. These groups were also among the lowest in life expectancy, often only thirty years. This was not due to the climates they endured because groups in similar climates who ate diets of little or no animal flesh had some of the highest life expectancies in the world.

World health statistics found that large numbers of Russian Caucasians, Yucatan Indians and East Indian Todas, and the Pakistan Hunzakuts have life expectancies of ninety to one hundred years!

The populations with the very longest life spans in the world are the Vilcambas, who reside in the Andes of Ecuador; the Abkhasians, who live on the Black Sea in the USSR; and the Hunzas, who live in the Himalayas of Northern Pakistan. These groups were discovered to have an astonishing similarity in their diets. All are either totally vegetarian or close to it. The Hunzas are the largest group of the three and eat almost no animal products whatsoever. Meat and dairy products together, account for only 1.5% of their total calories.

Researchers who visited these cultures found it interesting that the people not only enjoy such longevity, but they enjoy full, active lives throughout their many years. They show no signs of the many degenerative diseases that are common in our elderly population in the U.S. Said one researcher, "They work and play at eighty and beyond; most of those who reach their hundredth birthday continue to be active, and retirement is not heard of. The absence of meat (excess protein) in their diets causes slower growth and slim, compact body frames. With age, wisdom accumulates, but physical degeneration is limited so the senior citizens of these remote societies have something unique to contribute to the lives of others. They are revered."

Common Questions and Answers about Becoming a Vegetarian:

"What is a vegetarian?"

Generally speaking, a vegetarian is a person who does not eat meat, fowl, fish, or any by-product such as bone meal, animal fats, or gelatin. Vegetarians live on a diet of grains, pulses (peas, beans and lentils are known as pulses), nuts, seeds, vegetables, and fruit—some vegetarians eat eggs, milk, and milk products. Vegetarians who avoid all flesh and meat products, and eat only plant-based foods are called vegans.

It is a myth to think we need to "eat protein to get protein." If that was the case, where do cows get all the protein from, which they obviously have — seeing their huge bodies and the amount of protein that is supposed to be in the milk they give? Cows get their protein from the grass they eat. Green leafy vegetables have small quantities of very high-quality protein, and cows do eat a lot of grass.

The actual fact is that the protein of each animal is unique. Animal protein is different from human protein though both are made of amino acids. If you eat animal protein, the body needs to break it up into its component amino acids and then reassemble it as human protein. If you eat fresh fruits, you are getting the amino acids straight away and are saving the body the trouble of breaking the proteins up first.

Amino acids are present in almost all the foods we eat, even in strawberries, potatoes, or in rice, wheat, or lentils. It is very difficult for anyone who is eating three meals a day of an average diet (and I mean average, not a particularly healthy diet or a hygienic diet) to suffer from a protein deficiency. Even rice and dal or roti and vegetable (common Indian dishes) give us enough of the protein we need.

"Is it difficult being a vegetarian?"

Not at all. Vegetarian options are available in most grocery stores and many restaurants. Vegetarian food is easy to cook—many of your snack meals may already be vegetarian. And there are lots of delicious vegetarian recipes and vegetarian flavors to choose from. Once you move away from an animal-based diet, your body will be so much healthier!

"But is vegetarianism healthy?"

Yes. As long as you follow a balanced vegetarian diet, you'll be perfectly healthy. The truth is, a balanced vegetarian eating plan has significant health benefits over the Western meat-diet. That's why medical studies reveal time and again that vegetarians are less likely to suffer from such illnesses as heart disease, cancer, diet-related diabetes, obesity, and high blood pressure.

"Is vegetarian food as tasty as meat?"

Yes, it is! Remember, much of the "taste" we associate with meat is actually fat. And many instant or processed meat-foods are high in salt. So you're often tasting fat and salt—not the meat itself! Besides, a vegetarian meal doesn't mean taking the meat away and leaving the side vegetables. There are loads of different vegetarian tastes you can create from the hundreds of different vegetables, pastas, grains, fruit, pulses, nuts, and seeds that exist.

"I've been told that vegetarian diets lack vital nutrients, like protein."

A well-balanced vegetarian diet provides all the nutrients you need for good health. For example, adequate protein —

and the essential amino acids protein is comprised of — can be found in nuts, soy, tofu, vegetarian cheeses, as well as combinations of foods such as beans, peas, grains and almost all of the fresh fruit and vegetable foods. Even certain vegetables contain trace amounts of protein.

Health Benefits of a Vegetarian Diet

A vegetarian diet provides a wide range of health benefits. Research shows that vegetarians suffer less from many of the diseases associated with the typical Western diet, including obesity, coronary heart disease, hypertension, type II diabetes, diet-related cancers, diverticular disease, constipation and gall stones.

Vegetarian Diets Follow Dietary Guidelines

A typical vegetarian diet reflects most of the dietary recommendations for healthy eating, being low in saturated fat and high in fiber, complex carbohydrates, and fresh fruit and vegetables.

Vegetarian Diets Lower in Fat/Lipids

Vegetarian diets tend to be lower in total fat. Taber & Cook (1980) found lacto-ovo (eating dairy products and eggs) vegetarians to consume an average of 35% of energy as fat, compared to omnivores (meat eaters) consuming over 40% of

energy as fat. A study of the diets of a group of French vegetarians found they had a daily intake of 25% less fat than
non-vegetarians (Millet, 1989). Vegetarians also tend to eat
proportionally more polyunsaturated fat to saturated fat
compared with non-vegetarians. Animal products are the major
sources of dietary saturated fat.

Becoming a Vegetarian

There are no set rules to becoming a vegetarian. If you
wish, you can reduce your meat consumption gradually, or limit
yourself to fish only. Becoming a vegetarian can be a process,
not necessarily an overnight event! Some vegetarians would
say that vegetarianism is more of a way of life, not simply what
you put on your dinner plate.

Many teenagers try to become vegetarians overnight.
They think vegetarianism is "cool," but sometimes they lack the
patience to adapt their meat-eating habits to vegetarian ones
so they lose interest. The best way to move away from meat
and become a vegetarian is to take things gradually.

Becoming a Vegetarian – Some Tips

- Invest in a good vegetarian cookbook.

- Check out your local health food store—it's bound to have vegetarian foods and products you haven't seen before—and ask questions about vegetarian foods that are new to you.

- Buy vegetarian cheese. Some cheeses are still made with an ingredient from the stomachs of slaughtered calves, while vegetarian cheese uses vegetable-derived rennet. Many of the more unusual varieties such as Stilton and Brie are also now available in vegetarian versions.

- Buy legumes/pulses and lentils. No need to buy the dried variety — go for the canned or frozen types of kidney beans, garbanzo-beans (chick peas), etc.

- Make friends with soy products. Buy soybeans, try soymilk and experiment with tofu. You might prefer tofu in smoked varieties, but remember: it has no specific taste of its own — it's meant to absorb the flavor of other ingredients.

- Try TVP (textured vegetable protein) — buy the "flavored" variety and use it instead of ground beef in vegetarian lasagna, and other recipes.

  Start reading food labels. You'll be surprised how many non-meat foods contain meat-derivatives, like animal fats or gelatin.

A Basic Vegetarian Eating Plan

All the nutrients you need can quite easily be obtained from a vegetarian diet. And research shows that in many ways a vegetarian diet is healthier than that of a typical meat-eater. Nutrients are usually divided into macro-nutrients (carbohydrates, proteins, fats and oils), and micro-nutrients (vitamins and minerals). We also need regular fiber and six to eight glasses of water, per day.

As far as meal planning is concerned, here is a very rough guide to what you should eat every day on a balanced vegetarian diet.

- 4 or 5 servings of fruit and vegetables

- 3 or 4 servings of cereals/grains or potatoes

- 2 or 3 servings of legumes/pulses, nuts & seeds

- 2 servings of soy milk, soy or almond cheese, or other soy products

- A small amount of vegetable oil and margarine

- Some yeast extract, ideally fortified with vitamin B12.

How Important is Protein?

A lot of importance is traditionally given to protein in our diet. "Are you getting enough protein?" is something everyone seems to be worried about. People ask regularly "How do you get your protein if you don't eat any animal or dairy products?" The truth of the matter is that yes, protein is important. But so are carbohydrates. So are fats. So are vitamins, minerals and so on and so forth. Every part of the diet is important. And a deficiency (or excess) in any component will cause problems.

Human Protein Requirements

How much protein do we really need? It is not a simple question to answer because there are conflicting views. But one thing is clear; we need a lot less than previously thought. The U.S. Recommended Daily Allowance (RDA) for protein was over 100g per day per person not so long ago. It has been gradually reduced and currently, standards are about 52g for an average male and 44g for an average female. Actually there is a huge safety margin built into these numbers usually the actual requirements are ascertained and then doubled. This can be seen from the fact that the international standards (for the rest of the world's population) are 37g. for an average male and 29g for an average female. It is not logical that just because you are in the U.S. you need more protein than the rest of the world.

Amino Acid Pool Theory

Another theory you need to know about is the amino acid pool theory. Proteins are made up of amino acids and about twenty-three of them are known today. The body can synthesize fifteen of them from other things; only eight of them — called essential amino acids — need to be there in the food we eat. And guess which food has all these eight amino acids? Fresh fruit!

Dangers of Excessive Protein Consumption

Everyone knows of the dangers of excessive consumption of fats so people ask for lean meat and fish instead of red meat, etc. But very few know of the dangers of eating too much protein. Large amounts of animal protein contribute to osteoporosis, and kidney problems.

High protein diets are especially taxing to the liver and kidneys. When people eat too much protein, they take in more nitrogen than they need. This places a strain on the liver and kidneys, which must expel the extra nitrogen through urine.

Diets that are rich in protein, especially animal protein, are known to cause people to excrete more calcium than normal through their urine and increase the risk of osteoporosis. Countries with lower-protein diets have lower rates of osteoporosis and hip fractures.

Even heart disease, cancer, diabetes, arthritis, high choles-terol and other debilitating diseases have been linked to excessive protein consumption especially animal protein, which is naturally accompanied by high levels of saturated fat. Excessive amounts of saturated fat consumption in the diet have been linked to clogged arteries, low tissue oxygenation, slow metabo-lism, and heart and other degenerative diseases. Excess protein that is not used for building tissues or energy is converted by the liver and stored as fat in the body tissues. The links between animal protein and deteriorating health are numerous.

Our health depends on what we eat daily.

Foods are the building blocks of every cell in the body. Cells, the building blocks of our body, are responsible for the proper functioning of the whole body. Without adequate nutri-tion, we cannot expect ourselves to be healthy. The nutrition comes from what we eat and drink. It is important, therefore, to know what is good for our body and what is not.

Junk foods are empty calories.

These foods have little enzyme producing vitamins and minerals and contain a high level of calories. When we eat these empty calorie foods, the body is required to produce its own enzymes to convert these empty calories into usable energy. This is not an optimum scenario as enzyme-producing functions in our body should be reserved for the performance of vital metabolic reactions.

Given below are a list of junk (empty calorie) items that we should avoid. It is now up to you how you *can keep your four trillion cells happy.*

- Sugars and refined foods, like sugar and plain flour (maida)-based items like white bread and most packaged goods, like Twinkies and sugar donuts, etc.—Our body eventually turns sugars into fat. If you consume just 3 tsp of sugar daily, imagine how much sugar you would have consumed by the time you are 50 years of age, it will be about 275 kg, about 5 times your weight!

- Fats & Hydrogenated oils—They are found in cookies, chips, candy bars, fried foods, muffins, etc. etc. Remember there is nothing that is useful for our body in hydrogenated foods. The excessive fats stick to our arteries and cause the blockages leading to heart disease and strokes. They can also lead to cancer, arthritis, PMS and sexual dysfunction. Some fats, like Omega-3 fatty acids, are good for our bodies. (For more information about hydrogenated fats, read our fat and cholesterol page, Appendix 2.)

- High-carbohydrate foods—The primary cause of obesity in our society.

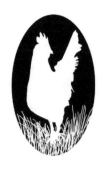

Conclusion

Let us start this loving awakening by understanding that our bodies are simply shelters for our souls. Our main purpose on this earth is to feed our souls and to worry less about feeding our bodies. To evolve and grow spiritually, and to have a loving relationship with God and our brothers and sisters who share this planet with us, including the animals. We are all connected through the spirit of God living within us. Isn't that alone reason for celebration. Life is wonderful because we have the Great Spirit living within us, and we cannot go wrong if we learn to listen to it!

Connecting to this life-giving source that unites all creation can be done in many ways. Meditate daily. Learn to listen to what your soul's purpose is here on earth. Learning and listening to what your soul already knows and what it has already chosen to do with your life is our true reason for walking this earth. Quieting the mind or what some experts call ego. That, I believe and have found in my spiritual journey, to be the single most difficult thing there is to do. The mind is a powerful tool, and a wonderful addition to our bodies, however, somewhere along the way, the mind took over what used to be our inner guide, our natural instincts , and our quiet listening. In our busy, everyday lives, we have lost contact with the quiet mission of our soul. The mind is so powerful that we don't even realize that it has taken over us. It is unable to live in the "now" that we should be dwelling in to truly enjoy this journey here on earth. It lives only in the past or the future. When the mind is in control, it is very difficult to enjoy the present. This happens to me quite a bit. I'm at a party, enjoying friends, food and drink, however, my mind wanders to what is happening tomorrow, or the next day, or a trip that I am going to take or whatever big event is coming or happening in the future. Or, a song will come on the radio, and poof, I am scooted back to another place and time, somewhere in the past. I started to notice this quite some time ago, and you will too if you just stop and listen to your thoughts. It's pretty amazing what you will realize. There are techniques to quiet the mind so that you can enjoy the moment and not dwell in places that keep you from truly enjoying life now. One book I found very helpful is *The Power of Now*, by Eckhart Tolle. This book set me on the right track in learning how to quiet the mind.

Walking in the forest or any kind of natural environment brings your soul back to life because we energize in those environments. Earth, trees, fire, and water are the most pure sources of good energy and essence. Being in the quiet natural environment of nature is a sure way to begin the healing process of quieting the mind/ego, which is the beginning to living your life in the love energy.

Conclusion

Join me in a wonderful pursuit: to spread love to everyone and everything we meet.

Bless you and please, love ALL of our animals, too!

Good luck to you on your journey!

Appendix 1
Food-borne Illnesses

Food-borne illness remains a serious, yet largely preventable, health threat. Each year in the United States food-borne illness accounts for 76 million sicknesses, 325,000 hospitalizations, and 5,000 deaths. Specifically, thousands of children die each year from the E. coli pathogen found in foods.

Recently, the television show *Dateline* did an exposé on public health entitled "Dirty Dining." It is pretty grim. Fast food is served fast, and you eat it fast, so you might not notice the restaurant is a little dirty. The fact is that no one had ever conducted a national survey looking at the cleanliness of fast food chains, until *Dateline's* report. Journalists took cameras undercover for the first-ever investigation on America's fast food chains. Are they clean and safe? Well, here's the bottom line: We're a nation fueled by fast food —burgers and fries, tacos, fried chicken. It's hot, tasty, and easy. And with millions and millions of "meals" sold every day, most of us just assume it's all clean and safe. But, when it's not, it can be devastating.

After eating at a McDonald's in Erwin, Tennessee, one hundred people became violently ill. Some ended up in the hospital, dehydrated, and even hallucinating. The Centers for Disease Control theorized ill employees may have contaminated food with a virus, although McDonald's disputes that.

Meanwhile, after eating at a KFC in Colorado, Gianni

Velotta was infected with a dangerous salmonella bacteria. His mother says he almost died. Natalle Velotta said, "His kidneys weren't working. I mean, there's just no words to explain how bad it actually was."

The biggest ten chains have 75,000 restaurants. *Dateline* couldn't check each one, so they chose one hundred of each chain, totaling one thousand. The following are some of the findings:

McDonald's: The golden arches came in after one hundred stores were inspected with 136 critical violations. Some didn't have trained and certified food handlers on the job (required in many states). The problem with that is you can't have people preparing food who don't know you can't combine raw meat with cooked meat, by people who don't understand the importance of proper temperatures in food preparation.

Subway: The one hundred Subways looked at totaled 160 critical violations. A recurring problem at the sandwich chain was improper food holding temperatures. Bacteria present in food that's already cooked can start to grow, and it can reach levels that can cause serious illness for the consumers.

Jack in the Box: They too had a total of 164 critical violations out of the one hundred visited. Jack in the Box in Ventura, California had several customer complaints of food-borne illness.

Wendys: One hundred Wendy's had 206 critical violations. That puts Wendy's number three in the *Dateline* dirty dining survey. At Wendy's in Mesa, Arizona, inspectors noticed repeated problems with food holding temperatures, mice droppings on the shelves, bare hand food contact, and one food-borne illness complaint.

Taco Bell: The one hundred Taco Bell's sampled, they had the fewest total critical violations, 91, making it the best performer in the *Dateline* survey. However, it was not without problems. Recurring violations included dirty food preparation counters and rodent droppings.

KFC: The one hundred KFC's sampled tallied up 157 critical violations, and two thirds of the "finger lickin'" good restaurants had at least one critical violation. Remember, it was at KFC the Health Department says, that little Gianni Velotta picked up salmonella poisoning last year. We've now learned that another child was also sickened there, and the same restaurant has since been cited for three more critical violations.

Then, *Dateline* collected and examined local health inspection reports for the last year and one half on each of these one thousand restaurants. Some were inspected just once, some more often, their findings may do more than surprise you. Some of the horror stories in *Dateline's* dirty dining survey just might turn your stomach.

In a Chicago Wendy's, inspectors found dead rodents decomposing on a rattrap. At a California Taco Bell, someone bit into a taco, only to find chewing gum. An inspector in Texas found a worm in a Wendy's salad. At a Hardee's in Florida, a customer was handed a cup of soda with blood dripping from it. There was blood on her change as well. The list goes on . . . A cockroach in someone's soda, a sharp metal object in a man's sandwich. But as disgusting as these things are, they are rare. Experts say the things you can't see can be even more hazardous . . .

Appendix 2
Fats and Cholesterol

Fat and Cholesterol

Healthy lifestyle changes such as exercising regularly and quitting smoking can reduce your risk of heart disease, but another important change is one in dietary habits. Reduction in certain types of fat and cholesterol are very important. Lipids are the fats that circulate in your blood stream. Two types of these fats that are closely watched by your physician are cholesterol and triglycerides. Cholesterol is a fat-like substance found only in animal products. The highest sources of cholesterol comes from organ meats (example: liver) and eggs, but other common sources are any type of meat, poultry, cheese, and butterfat. Americans currently consume 400–500 milligrams of cholesterol a day, but the recommended amount is only 300 mg per day for the average person. By changing your eating pattern you can reduce your fat intake to the recommended level of not exceeding 30% of your daily calories.

Cholesterol—Good and Bad:

Cholesterol is essential for life to make strong cell

membranes and hormones. The body manufactures about 1,000 mgs of cholesterol daily. Too much cholesterol can cause fatty plaques on arterial walls which narrows the artery. This condition is known as atherosclerosis. The build up of fat on the vessel walls can occlude and in some case totally block the flow of blood to organs like the heart. When atherosclerosis occurs in heart vessels, also known as coronary heart disease, chest pain and heart attacks can result. The method of cholesterol transport in the blood separates cholesterol into "good" and "bad" types. The harmful type of cholesterol is known as low-density lipoproteins (LDL's). Lipoprotein is a combination of fat (lipo) and protein. LDL's are the most common type of cholesterol in your blood stream and are known as bad cholesterol because excessive amounts of this lipoprotein stick to vessel walls forming plaques. High density lipoproteins (HDL's) are known as good cholesterol because high levels of HDL's are associated with a reduced risk of heart disease. HDL's unstick LDL's from vessel walls and transport cholesterol out of the arteries.

Diet and Cholesterol

Your fat intake should not exceed 30% of your daily calories. There are two main types of fats which you may have read about. Saturated fats tend to increase your LDL's and are found mostly in animal products. These fats are solid at room temperature. Two vegetable oils are high in saturated fats and should be avoided, palm and coconut oil. To reduce the amount of saturated fat, cut back on items such as butter, lard, and cheese.

Appendix 2: Fats and Cholesterol

Polyunsaturated fats such as corn, soy, sunflower, and safflower oils reduce the amount of LDL's but also reduce the amount of HDL's in your blood. Polyunsaturated fats remain liquid at room temperature. The best fats to use are monounsaturated fats from peanut oil, canola oil, or olive oil which reduce LDL's but do not reduce the "good" HDL's.

A single egg yolk contains 250 mg of cholesterol, which is about the maximum daily intake recommended (300 mg) and eggs are high in fat. Thus the best recommendation on eggs is to use them in moderation and where possible use an egg white product as an egg substitute. Try to limit egg consumption to approximately three a week in all items you eat (including baked goods).

Try to bake, broil, steam, microwave or poach your foods and avoid fried foods. Use vegetable cooking sprays instead of greasing pans. For protein in your diet — and the essential amino acids which protein is comprised of — eat more soy products, peas and beans. The following are known to contain all eight essential amino acids needed from food: carrots, brussel sprouts, cabbage, cauliflower, corn, cucumbers, eggplant, kale, okra, potatoes, summer squash, sweet potatoes, tomatoes and bananas. To reduce fat in dairy foods, use soy milk or soy yogurt. Try the reduced fat cheese and when possible look for the cheeses made with soy or almond. Whole grains in breads, cereals, and pastas are a good choice. Oatmeal and oatbran is a good choice since it appears to have some cholesterol lowering effect. be sure to read any commercial baked products carefully since many may be prepared with the "bad" oils such as palm or coconut. Eat all of the fruits and vegetables you want. They are naturally low in saturated fat, but avoid avocados and coconuts which are exceptions to the rule.

When eating out avoid fast food chains and be sure to look for heart healthy items on the menu. Do not be afraid to ask how an item is prepared and ask if changes are possible to make it healthier for you. Most restaurants are becoming aware of the need for heart healthy items and if one refuses your request, consider eating somewhere else. Remember you are the customer.

These are general guidelines which can help you to a healthier lifestyle.

Appendix 3
References

2003–2004 Naples Daily News, Naples, FL

2004 The Doctor's Medical Library, Food Myths

American Cancer Society: Nutrition & Cancer

The Center for Science in the Public Interest

CaringConsumer.com—A Guide to Living Kindly (PETA)

Columbia Daily Tribune: "America's Growing Numbers, Fast Food & Obesity."

Dateline NBC: MSNBC News: Consumer Alert

Entrepreneur.com: "Franchize Zone, The future of Fast Food, Part 1"

Factory Farming: www.factoryfarming.org

Farm Sanctuary: www.farmsanctuary.org

Farm Sanctuary's Sentient Beings: www.sentientbeings.org

Food & Drug Administration (FDA)

Federal Trade Commission (FTC): "For the Consumer"

First Food/First Institute for Food and Development Policy

Gross, Daniel: "Unhappy meal: What's Wrong with Burger King?" (slate.msn.com; 06/24/04)

International Vegetarian Union: www.ivu.org

Lyman, Howard F.: *Mad Cowboy: Plain Truth from the Cattle Rancher Who Won't Eat Meat* (Voice for a Viable Future; ISBN: 0-684-84516-4)

MarketResearch.com

People for the Ethical Treatment of Animals (PETA): www.peta.org

Masson, Jeffrey, *The Pig Who Sang to the Moon: The Emotional World of Farm Animals* (Ballantine Books, ISBN 034545281X)

Medterms.com

The National Restaurant Association

Nutrifit, LLC: www.nutrifitonline.com

Organic Consumers Association: www.organicconsumers.org

Pelman V McDonald's: Health Law Perspectives/Obesity.

Preferred Care: Health Centers, "Do you want that supersized?"

Robbins, John, *Diet for a New America: How Your Food Choices Affect Your Health, Happiness and the Future of Life on Earth* (H. J. Kramer, ISBN 0915811812)

The Robert Wood Johnson Foundation: Pubic Health Leadership and capacity.

United Poultry Concerns: upc-online.org

Usborne, David: "Film records effects of eating only McDonald's for a month," (01/25/04)

U.S. Department of Agriculture (USDA)

Vartan, Starre: "Want Cancer With That?," AlterNet

Vegetarian Diet Information 2003–2004

Vegetarians International Voice for Animals (VIVA!): www.viva.org.uk

World Health Organization (WHO)

Web Sites:

If you are interested in helping fight cruelty to animals, please visit the following sites:

AdoptATurkey.org

BanCruelFarms.org

coc.net (Compassion over Killing)

www.compassionoverkilling.org

FactoryFarming.com
farmsanctary.org
farmanimalshelters.org
FreeFarmAnimals.org
hsus.org/ace/15419
IVU.org
www.mercyforanimals.org
NJFarms.org
NoDowners.org
NoFoieGras.org
NoVeal.org
peta.org
Poultry.org
SentientBeings.org
taosanctuaries.org/about/index.htm
upc-online.org
VegForLife.org
WalkForFarmAnimals.org

Additional Resources:

Black Beauty Ranch, in Murchison, TX:
    www.blackbeautyranch.org
Farm Sanctuary, with sanctuaries in Orland, California and
    Watkins Glen, New York: www.farmsanctuary.org
Greenpeople Sanctuary. In many many states in U.S. and
    Canada: .greenpeople.org/sanctuary.htmSanctuaries.
Poplar Springs Animals Sanctuary, in Poolsville, MD:
    www.animalsanctuary.org
Sanctuaries. This site lists the best and most trusted animal
    sanctuaries: www.sanctuaries.org
Wilderness Ranch, in Loveland, Colorado:
    www.wildernessranch.org

Book References:

Bauston, Gene, *Battered Birds, Crated Herds: How we Treat the Animals We Eat* (Watkins Glen, NY: Farm Sanctuary: 1996)

Davis, Karen: *More than a meal: The Turkey in History, Myth, Ritual, and Reality:* (New York, Lantern Books, 2001) *Prisoned Chickens Poisoned Eggs, An Inside Look at the Modern Poultry Industry* (Summertown, TN Book Publishing Company, 1996).

Ehret, Prof. Arnold, *Rational Fasting, for Physical, Mental, Spiritual Rejuvenation*: *Mucusless Diet Healing System, Scientific Method of Eating Your Way to Health* (Ehret Literature Publishing Co., 1975, 1953)

Giehl, Dudley, *Vegetarianism: A Way of Life* (New York, Barns & Noble, 1979)

Hausman, Patricia and Hurley, Judeth: *The Healing Foods, The Ultimate Authority on the Curative Power of Nutrition* (Rodale Press, 1989)

Lappe', Francis Moore, *Diet for a Small Planet* (New York, Ballantine Books, 1987)

Lyman, Howard F., with Glen Merzer: *Mad Cowboy: Plain Truth from the Cattle Rancher Who Won't Eat Meat* (New York, Scribner, 1998)

Malkmus, Rhonda, *Recipies for Life: From God's Garden*

Mason, Jim and Peter Singer, *Animal Factories* (New York Harmony Books, 1990)

Masson, Jeffrey: *The Pig Who Sang to the Moon, The Emotional World of Farm Animals* (The Random House Publishing Group, 2003)

Nestle, Marion, *Food Politics: How the Food Industry Influences Nutrition and Health* (Berkeley: University of

California Press, 2002)

Robbins, John, *Diet for a New America, How Your Food Choices Affect Your Health, Happiness, and the Future of Life on Earth* (H. J. Kramer, Inc., 1987)

Regan, Tom: *Empty Cages: Facing the Challenge of Animal Rights* (Rowman & Littlefield Publishers, 2004)

Scully, Matthew, *Dominion: The Power of Man, the Suffering of Animals, and the Call to Mercy* (St. Martin's Press, NY, 2002)

Singer, Pete: *Animal Liberation* (Harper Collins Publishing, NY, 2002)

Sunstein, Cass R. and Nussbaum, Martha Craven : *Animal Rights: Current Debates and New Directions* (Oxford University Press, 2004)

Sussman, Vic, *The Vegetarian Alternative: A Guide to a Healthful and Humane Diet* (Rodale Press, Emmaus, PA, 1978)

Wise, Steven M: *Rattling the Cage: Towards Legal Rights for Animals:* (Perseus Books, NY, 1999)

Free Vegetarian Starter Kit

PETA offers a free "Vegetarian Starter Kit" featuring recipes, tips, and ideas to get you started. To obtain your kit, visit www.vegetarianstarterkit.com.

Also visit www.vegforlife.org for a free *Guide to Vegetarian Living* from Farm Sanctuary.

Vegan/Vegetarian Cookbooks:

20 Minutes to Dinner, (Grogan)

Almost No-Fat Cookbook, The (Grogan)

American Vegetarian Cookbook, The (Diamond)

Angel Foods, (Soria)
Being Vegetarian, (Havala)
Best in the World, The (Barnard)
Compassionate Cook, The (Newkirk)
Conscious Eating, (Cousens)
Convenient Vegetarian, The (Messina)
Cooking Vegetarian, (Melina)
Dining in the Raw, (Romano)
Dr. Dean Ornish's Program for Reversing Heart Disease, (Ornish)
Fat-Free & Easy, (Raymond)
Food For Life, (Barnard)
Foods That Fight Pain, (Barnard)
Good Life, The (Nearing)
Health Promoting Cookbook, The (Goldhamer)
How It All Vegan!, (Kramer)
Incredibly Delicious, (World)
Japanese Cooking, (Schinner)
Millennium Cookbook, The (Tucker)
New Farm Cookbook, The (Hagler)
New Vegetarian Baby, (Yntema)
Nonna's Italian Kitchen, (Grogan)
Peaceful Palate, The (Raymond)
Raw: The Uncook Book, (Juliano)
Shopping Guide for Caring Consumers — 2000, (PeTA)
Soup's On!, (Bloomfield)
Soyfoods Cooking for a Positive Menopause, (Grogan)
Sproutman's Kitchen Garden Cookbook, (Meyerowitz)
Sprouts: The Miracle Food, (Meyerowitz)
Sweet and Natural, (McCarty)

Tofu Tollbooth, (Zipern)
Vegetarian Cooking for People with Allergies, (Rettner)
Vegetarian Magic, (Nowakowski)
Vegetarian Way, The (Messina)
You Can Save the Animals, (Newkirk)

Shopping at the PETA Mall

This online shopping mall is directed at the caring consumer and features animal-friendly apparel, cruelty-free gifts, health and beauty essentials tested on people (not animals), vegan foods from around the world, and more. A percentage of purchases benefit PETA.

Magazines

Vegetarian Times: vegetariantimes.com
Natural Health: naturalhealth.com
Veggie Life: www.veggielife.com
VegNews: www.vegnews.com

Appendix 4
Famous Vegetarians/Vegans

ACTORS

Affleck, Casey
Aherne, Caroline
Anderson, Gillian
Anglehart, Raynald
Arthur, Bea
Astin, John
Bach, Richard & Leslie
Baldwin, Alec
Bardot, Brigitte
Barrymore, Drew
Basinger, Kim
Baxter, Meredith
Benedict, Dirk
Benson, Amber
Berkley, Elizabeth
Bingham, Traci
Birch, Thora
Bloom, Orlando ??
Bogdanovich, Peter
Briers, Lucy
Brown, "Downtown" Julie
Bubbles
Burstyn, Ellen
Butler, Brett
Cameron, Kirk
Cauffiel, Jessica
Cinnamon, Cindy
Clarke, Margi
Cleese, John
Conant, Sean
Cook, Racheal Leigh
Corbett, John

Cromwell, James
Cruz, Penelope
Cush, Sandra
Dafoe, Willem
Danson, Ted
DeVito, Danny
Diaz, Cameron
DiCaprio, Leonardo
Duchovny, David
Elise, Christine
Ferris, Pam
Fox, Jorja
Fox, Michael J.
Frost, Sadie
Furlong, Edward
Garofalo, Janeane
Garth, Jennie
Gere Richard
Gielgud, Sir John
Gunter, Bob
Harper, Valerie
Harrelson, Woody
Hartnett, Josh
Hawthorne, Nigel
Hemmingway, Mariel
Henner, Marlu
Hoffmann, Dustin
Holmes, Katie
Imbruglia, Natalie
Jennings, Kevin Robert
Judd, Ashley
Kemp, Martin
Kennedy, Gerard

Keymah, T'Keyah Crystal
Law, Jude
Leachman, Cloris
Lenk, Tom
Lennon, Jarrett
Louis-Dreyfus, Julia
Love, Willamina
Lumley, Joanna
Maguire, Tobey
Marcil, Vanessa
Martin, Steve
Martin, Ty Mathis, Samantha
McClanahan, Rue
Mckellen, Sir Ian
Milligan, Spike
Mills, Hayley
Moore, Demi
Morales, Esai
Murphy, Brittany
Nealon, Kevin & Linda
Newman, Paul
Paltrow, Gwyneth
Paquin, Anna
Paul, Alexandra
Pearce, Guy
Peterson, Cassandra
Phoenix, Joaquin
Phoenix, Rain
Phoenix, Summer
Pitt, Brad
Plimpton, Martha
Portman, Natalie
Powers, Stephanie
Raven, Robin
Regalbuto, Joe
Roache, Linus
Roberts, Julia
Sawalha, Julia
Seagal, Steven
Sellers, Peter

Shaw, Martin
Shields Brooke
Silverstone, Alicia
Simpson, Lisa
Stamp, Terence
Stiles, Julia
Stoltz, Er Ðic
Stoner, Lynda
Sumner, Peter
T! Alexander
Talbert, Jonathan Tristan
Thiessen, Tiffani-Amber
Thomas, Jonathan Taylor
Tyler, Liv
Tyler-Moore, Mary
Ventimiglia, Milo
Vaughn, Vince
Wagner, Kristina
Wagner, Lindsay
Watts, Naomi
Weaver, Dennis
Winslet, Kate
Witherspoon, Reese

TV PERSONALITIES

Adams, Kaye
Armstrong, Pamela
Barker, Bob
Carling, Julia
Cool, Phil
Cotton, Fearne
Drucker, Michel
Engelke, Anke
Eubanks, Kevin
Forrester, Philippa
G, Andrew
Groothuizen, Angela
Hamburger, Neil
Hertsenberg, Antoinette
Holt, Viola

Appendix 4: Famous Vegetarians/Vegans

Jordan, Diane Louise
Kelder , Jord
Lake, Ricki
Landini, Tina
Maher, Bill
Martin, Paul
Miller, Nick
Osbourne, Kelly
Red Ronnie
Roberts, Julia
Rogers, Fred
Seinfeld, Jerry
Simpson, Lisa
Snyder, Julie
Sperling, Sy
Strachan, Michaela
Thomas, Jonathan Taylor
Turner, Anthea
Turner, Wendy
Tyler Moore, Mary
Wood, Victoria
Wai Lana

**ADDITIONAL
CELEBRITIES:**
Abboit, Nick
Blackburn, Tony
Brooks, Hildi
Casey Kasem
Eligon, Ian D' Goose
Free, Louie
Greening, Kevin
Griffin, Meg
Imus, Don
Jackie O
Mitchell, Chris
Peel, John
Riley, Marc
Robert, Pierre
Scott, Rik

Skinner, Nancy
Sullivan, Sarah
Travis, Dave Lee
Visage, Michelle
Walden, Shelton
Walker, Jonny,
Wilkes-Johnson, Shirley

**FASHION: MODELS, DESIGNERS,
PHOTOGRAPHERS**
Alt, Carol
Amini, Elizabeth
Auermann, Nadja
Bailey, David
Blyth, Jenny
Bordes, Pamela
Brinkley, Christie
Cooper, Victoria
Garley, Rachael
Hill, Angie
Le Bon, Yasmin
Linthout, Marieken
Lloyd, Kathy
McCartney, Stella
McKenna, Gail
Messenger, Melinda
Moss, Kate
Otis, Carre
Patitz, Tatjana
Schenkenbach, Gabriela
Scherrer, Laetizia
Stone, Christine
Turlington, Christy
Valentina

**FAMOUS MUSICIANS:
ROCK & POP**
Abram, Tom
Adams, Bryan
AFI

Albarn, Damon
Ament, Jeff
Amorrossi, Vanessa
Anderson, Brett
Anderson, Jon
Apple, Fiona
Arco Iris
Armstrong, Billie Joe
B52s
Badu, Erykah
Barlow, Gary
Barre, Martin
Barrett, Bucky
Beatz, J
Beck Jeff
Beck, Roscoe
Beloved Binge
Beltramo-Shay, Andi
Blalock, Gene
Blur
Bolan, Marc
Bolton, Michael
Bono
Boston
Bowers, Chris
Boy George
Boyd, Brandon
Brandy
Burchill, Charlie
Burke, Clem
Burrow, Brian
Bush, Kate
Butler, Bernard
Butler, Biff
Campbell, Vivian
Carcass
Carlisle, Belinda
Chalk, Matthew
Clayden, J.S.
Cobain, Kurt

Codling, Neil
Cody, Jessica
Coffey, Jefferey S. "King"
Cole Paula
Collen Phil
Dale, Dick
Dangers, Jack
Davies, Ray & Dav
Deakin, Douglas
Delp, Brad
Dennis, Cathy
Depeche Mode
Donots
Eighty-Six
Etheridge, Melissa
Feldmann, John
Franti, Michael
French, Sally
Frischman, Justine
Froese, Edgar
G-7 Welcoming Committee Records
Gabriel, Peter
Gentille, Linda
Gibb, Barry
Gibb, Robin
Gordon, Mike
Green, Derrick
Greenwald, Alex
Greenway, Barney
Hakim, Omar
Hammett, Kirk
Hamill, Christopher
Hammond, Marie-Lynn
Hariharan, Vijay
Hatfield, Julianna
Harlow, Leah
Harrison, George
Haslam, Annie
Hayes, Darren
Hetfield, James

Appendix 4: Famous Vegetarians/Vegans

Houston, Whitney
Howe, Steve
Hurst, James
Hynde, Chrissie
Idol, Billy
Ildjarn
Incubus
India.Arie
Jackson, Eddie
Jackson, Michael
Jett, Joan
Jocz , Steve
Johansson, Richard
Johns, Daniel
Johnson, Eric
Jones, Howard
Jorgenson, John
Jovanotti
Kallio, Santeri
Kerr, Jim
Kiedis, Anthony
Kowalczyk, Edward
Kravitz, Lenny
Kula Shaker
Laine, Olli-Pekka "Oppu"
Lang, K.D.
Lange, Robert John"Mutt"
Lavigne, Avril
Lee, Jon from Sclub7
Leigh-Chantelle
Lenchantin, Paz
Lennon, John and Yoko
Loeb, Lisa
Luca, Martello
Madonna
Marr, Johnny
Marshall, Steve
Martin, Billy
Martin, Ricky
May, Brian

McCartney, James
McCartney, Paul and Linda
Mclachlan, Sarah
McRe ćynolds, Ryan
Meatloaf
Mel C
Mendel, Nate
Merchant, Natalie
Mey, Reinhard
Minogue, Dannii
Moby
Moore, Christie
Mae Moore
Miles, Ellen
Molina, Pablo
Morissette, Alanis
Morrissey
Morse, Steve
Mullen Junior, Larry
Munter, Rose and Hamlin, Faye
Naked, Bif
Namubiru, Olivia
Nekro
Nico
Nova, Heather
Nya
O'Riordan, Dolores
Oberst, Conor
Owen, Mark
Perry, Steve
Pertusi, Ciro
Pink
Phoenix, River
Prince
Rage Against the Machine
Ramone, Joey
Rhodes, Nick
Rockett, Rikki
Rodriguez-Lopez, Omar
Safka, Melanie

Savor, Doug
Scholz, Tom
Schwartzman, Jason
Scilipoti, Antonietta
Shelter
Shiflett, Chris
Sines, Todd
Sioux, Siouxsie
Skinny Puppy
Sky, Bobby
Slick, Grace
Smith, Robert
Smiths, The
Spears, Britney
Starr, Ringo
Static, Wayne
Sting
Stipe, Michael
Tankian, Serj
Taylor, Ben
Timberlake, Justin
The Used, Quinn Allman
Thompson, Richard
Thumb (the whole band)
Tiller, Felicia
Tootsie
Turner, Tina
TV Smith
Twain, Shania
Urlaub, Farin
Vai, Steve
van Zalm, Peggy
Vedder, Eddie
Ward, Bill
Way, Pete
Weir, Bob
Welty Ron
Wiedlin, Jane
Williams, Vanessa
Williams, Wendy O.
Wray, Link

Yankovic, "Weird" Al
Yorke, Thom
Zanella, Santiago
Zappa - Dweezil, Moon, Ahmet, Diva
Zavala, Cedric Bixler

MUSICIANS: JAZZ, BLUES, COUNTRY, FOLK
Baez, Joan
Butler, John
Caballe, Montserrat
Cage, John,
Cohen, Leonard
Davies, Rick, and Sytek, Jane (Sytek and Davies),
Dickson, Barbara
Dylan, Bob
Holst , Gustav
Jonas, Peter
McPhee, Tony
Menuhin, Yehudi
Mullova, Viktoria
Musselwhite, Charlie
Paterson, Rober
Paterson,Victoria
Safka, Melanie
Sanders, Ric
Sharp, Cecil
Twain, Shania
Wagner, Richard
Yoakum, Dwigh

POLITICIANS, STATESPERSONS, ACTIVISTS AND BUSINESS PEOPLE:
Abourezk, James G.
Advani, L.K.
Anthony, Susan B
Bhandari, Shri. Sunder Singh
Banks, Tony, MP
Bartlett, Andrew

Appendix 4: Famous Vegetarians/Vegans

Barton, Clara
Benn, Tony
Braun, Nathan
Campbell, Anne
Chailert, Sangduen (Lek)
Chang, Yung-fa
Chavez, Cesar
Clarke, Alan
Clinton, Chelsea
Cohen, Harry
Craigavon, Viscount
Cripps, Sir Stafford
Das, Radha Krishna
Desai, Morarj
Dinshah, H.Jay
Lord Dowding
Lady Dowding
Drees, Willem
Erskine, Lord
Fischer, Joschka
Franklin, Benjamin
Gandhi, Maneka
Gandhi, Mohandas Karamchand
Gilman, Anne
Gompertz, Lewi
Gregory, Dick
Gwyther, Christine
Hill, Julia "Butterfly"
Hitler, Adolf
Jacobs, Andrew
Jefferson, Thomas
Jobs, Steve
Junblatt, Kamel
Kane, Rose
Kaufman, Ron
Kaunda, Dr. Kenneth David Buchizya
Kostov, Ivan
Kucinich, Dennis
Leuenberger, Moritz
Lutz, Robert

Lyman, Howard
Mankar, Sri Jayantilal N
Marijke, Vos
Masire, Sir Q. K. J.
Merchant, i Piers
Mokhiber, Alber
More, Sir Thomas
Nearing, Helen
Nearing, Scott
Ohlsson, Birgitta
Paine, Thomas
Patel, Sardar Vallabhbhai
Pick, Philip L.
Rajagopalachary, Chakravarthy
Rao, P.V. Narasimha
Shastri, Lal Bhadur
Sof'a of Greece
Spencer, Graham
Vajpayi, atal bihari
Weatherall, Bernard

SPORTS PERSONALITIES:
Aaron, Hank
Badman, Natascha
Bennett, Michael
Bird, Larry
Boyer, Jonathan
Brock, Peter
Burfoot, Amby
Burnquist, Bob
Burwash, Pete
Cahling, Andreas
Chappell, Greg
Cope, Simon
De Costella, Robert
Earle, Robbie
Evert, Christine
Goldberg, Bill
Gray, Estelle
Heidrich, Dr.Ruth

133

Hellriegel, Thomas
Hepburn, Doug
Hilligenn, Roy
Holmes, Keith
Howard, Desmond
Jurek, Scott
Kaat, Jim
Kalbermatten, Frederik
King, Billie Jean
Kowalski, Killer
Kumble, Anil
LaLonde, Donnie
LaRussa, Tony
Laumann, Silken
Lee, Bruce
Lewis, Carl
Linares, Sixto
Lynn, Jamie
Los Dolares
Males, Dan
Marek, Cheryl
Mihelich, Taj
MŸller, Nicolas
Monbiot, Katherine
Moses, Ed
MŸller, Jutta
Nava, Ricardo Torres
Navratilova, Martina
Niewiek, Julie Ann
Nurmi, Paavo
Oakes, Fiona
Osborn, Tom
Parish, Rober
Pearl, Bill
Peeler, Anthony
Roa, Roa
Rowley, Geoff
Ryde, Dr David
Sanderson, Danielle
Scott, Dave

Spaeth-Herring, Debbie
Sumners, Rosalyn
Thomas, Jamie
Vaughn, Jacques
Vialli, Gianluca
Walton, Bill
Watson, Emmil
Williams, Serena

WRITERS, ARTISTS AND PHILOSOPHERS:
Adams, Scott
Alcott, Louisa May
Anthony, Piers
Arnold, Sir Edwin
Barker, Clive
Bass, Jules
Bentham, Jeremy
Berry, Rynn
Breathed, Berke
Brewer, Gene
Borges, Boris
Bronte, Charlotte
Bush, Wilhelm
Byron, Lord (George Gordon)
Clark, Stephen
Coe, Sue
Coetzee, J. M.
Conant, Todd
Confucius
da Vinci, Leonardo
Diamond, Marilyn
Ensler, Eve
Gach, Gary
Goldsmith, Oliver
Gross-Foster, Karen
Guatemala, Alberto Chavez
Ha, Peter
Hardin, Valerie
Hood, Thomas

Howard-Johnson, Carolyn
Hughs, Ted
Ihomocl, Mutaka
Kafka, Franz
Kaplan, Helmut F.
Lane, Carla
Lappe, Frances Moore
Mayson, John
McGinn, Colin
Milligan, Spike
Mandeville, Bernard de
Mehta, Alka
Midgley, Mary
Montaigne, Michel Eyquem de
Naipaul, V.S
Newton, John Frank
Plato
Reclus, Elis e
Redfield, James
Regan, Tom
Rendell, Ruth
Rifkin, Jeremy
Ritson, Joseph
Robbins, Anthony
Robbins, John
Roth, Geneen
Salt, Henry
Sanminiatelli, Bino
Sarma, Seshendra
Schne oll, Donald
Shaw, George Bernard
Schirneck, Hubert
Schwartz, Richard
Shankar, Sri Sri Ravi
Shelley, Mary Wolstonecraft
Shelley, Percy Bysshe
Singer Isaac Bashevis
Singer, Professor Peter
Southey, Robert
Spencer, Colin

Theroux, Paul
Thomas, Dilip
Thoreau, Henry David
Thiruvalluvar
Thomas, Rev.Dr. Donald
Tolstoy, Leo Nikolayevich
Tryon, Thomas
Voltaire
Walker, Alice
Wynne-Tyson, Jon
Zephaniah, Benjamin

**SCIENTISTS, PHYSICIANS &
HEALTHCARE PROFESSIONALS:**
Appleby, Paul
Attwood, Charles, M.D
Babcock, Dr Andrew
Bajaj, Prof. (Dr.) Madan Mohan
Barnard, Neal, M.D.
Bravo, Dr. Arturo Alvarez
Borenstein, Nathaniel
Campbell, T. Colin, Ph.D
Chawla, Dr. Kalpana
Cheyne, George
Chiewsilp, Dumrong , M.D., M.P.H.
Coxeter, Donald
da Vinci, Leonardo
Diehl, Hans, Dr. Hsc.
Dunn , Prof. Floyd W.
Edison, Thomas A.
Einstein, Albert
Fuhrman, Joel H. MD
Gassendi, Pierre
Goodall, Jane
Graham , Dr Douglas
Greene, Professor Brian
Greger, Michael
Gruben , Professor Rosalind
Ha, Peter (Ha Phuoc Thao)
Hartley, David

Heidrich, Ruth, PhD
Heimlich, Henry, M.D
Hershaft, Alex, PhD
Hood, Sandra
Jacobs, Brian
Jain, Dr.P.K.
Kakimoto, Dr Mitsuru,
    D.D.Sc.,Ph.D.,M.S.A
Kalam, A P J Abdul
Kingsford, Anna M.D
Klaper, Michael, M.D.
Kothavade , Dr. Rajendra J,
Latto, Dr. Gordon
Lacey, Professor Richard
Leclerc, George Louis , Comte de
    Buffon
Leitzmann, Prof.Dr.Claus
LeRoy , Bob MS, EdM
Lin, Robert I-San, Ph.D., CNS, FICN
Medkova, Irena Ph.D., MD
Melina, Vesanto
Monod, Pr Th odore
Morakote, Nimit, Ph.D.
McDougall, John, M.D.
Nickolayev, Prof. Yury
Oldfield , Dr.Josiah MA, DCL, MRCS,
    LRCP
Ornish MD, Dean
Pawaradhisan, Sudhisak
Pasquini, Claude PhD.
Phillips, Sir Richard
Rads, Prof.
Ramanujan, Srinivasa
Ray, John
Schainholz, Daníiel, MD
Schweitzer, Dr Albert
Singh, Dr Vijay Raj
Sirichotrat, Dr. Nithat
Spock, Benjamin
Suttajit, Maitree, Ph.D.,
Suttajit, Prof Siriwan

Tesla, Nikola
Tovivich, Dr. Phichai
Walsh, Stephen, PhD
Witten, Edward

RELIGIOUS LEADERS & MYSTICS:
Agnon, Shmuel Yosef
Amritanandamayi, Mata
Besant, Annie
Booth, General William
Dalai Lama of Tibet, His Holiness
    the XIV
Ferrier, Rev. John Todd
Fuchs, Stephen
Graham, Sylvester
Gross-Foster, Karen
Jesus & the early Christians
Krishnamurti, Jiddu
Krishna, Anand
Linzey, Rev.Dr.Andrew
Maimonedes (Rabbi Moses ben
    Maimon)
Maharishi Dayanand Saraswati
Maitreya
Metcalfe, Rev.William
Prabhupada, A.C. Bhaktivedanta
    Swami
Rajneesh, Bagwan Sri (Osho)
Raynaud de la Ferrire, Serge
Sathya Sai Baba
Shankar, Sri Sri Ravi
St Brendan
St.Francis of Assisi
Swedenborg, Emanuel
Thich Nhat Hanh
Wesley, John,
White, Ellen G
Whitworth, Maria
Yogananda, Paramahansa
Yogi, Maharishi Mahesh

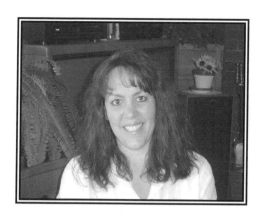

About the Author

Tina Volpe was raised in Lake View Terrace, California, a northern horsy suburb of Los Angeles. As a child, Volpe's home included many farm animals, most of which were eventually slaughtered for food for the family. This birth–life–death cycle had a huge affect on the author due to the love and friendship she felt with these creatures who, once living a comfortable life, were later served at the dinner table.

As a result of her love for, and interaction with, animals, Volpe became a vegetarian nearly three decades ago. Over the past five years, she has been studying the farm industry and the affects its business decisions and resulting procedures have on animals. Volpe also realized that the Fast Food Giants are a large cause of this suffering. This research convinced her that while advocacy groups have made advances in informing the public about farm industry carelessness, their efforts were not enough since animals are still suffering at the hand of businesses.

Tina Volpe is a member of, and has made contributions to, the many organizations that promote animal rights. She lives with her fiancé, Brian, in a small canyon cottage, about two miles from the house where she was raised.

Order Form

Quantity		Total
_____	**The Fast Food Craze:** $ 13.95	____
	Wreaking Havoc on Our Bodies and Our Animals	

Subtotal	____
CA residents add sales tax	____
Shipping	____

($3.95 for the first book and $2.00 for each additional book)

TOTAL ENCLOSED   ____

This order form is for shipping within the United States only.

To order *The Fast Food Craze* shipped to Canada, the U.K., or Australia, visit www.BookSurge.com.

Mail this form and your check or money order to:

Canyon Publishing, LLC
12617 Trail Two
Kagel Canyon, CA 91342

Name:_____

Street:_____

City:_____State:_____ ZIP:_____

E-mail: _____

Thank you for your order.

Please allow two weeks for delivery.
Questions? Contact books@fastfoodcraze.com.

To order by credit card, visit www.fastfoodcraze.com.
Bookstores and not-for-profits, contact the publisher for discounts.
Phone: 818/899/5559 Fax: 818/899-3686